Allergy prevention for kids

Allergy prevention for kids

a nutritional guide

Dr Leo Galland

First published 1989

This edition produced for Parragon Books 1994

Copyright © 1988 Copestone Press
Additional Material © Bloomsbury Publishing Ltd.

British Library Cataloguing in Publication Data

A CIP catalogue record for this book
is available from the British Library

ISBN 185813885X

10 9 8 7 6 5 4 3 2 1

Typeset by Rowland Phototypesetting Ltd,
Bury St Edmunds, Suffolk
Printed in Britain by
HarperCollins Manufacturing, Glasgow

Dedicated with love and appreciation to my family: Chris, Nicole, Jeff, Jonathan, Christopher and Jordan. I never stop learning from each of you.

A note to the reader: The ideas, procedures and suggestions contained in this book are not intended as a substitute for consulting with your own doctor. All matters regarding your health require medical supervision.

Great thanks to Signe Hammer for her help in editing the manuscript, to Carol Nostrand for her help in preparing and testing the recipes, and to Sid Baker for his wisdom and clinical pearls.

Contents

Foreword

I am proud to write the foreword to this distinguished book because I consider it to represent the wave of the future. Certainly it is a clarion call for better nutrition for all our children. I truly believe that if even a modest number of people would follow its suggestions, we would have a healthier and happier population.

Parents today are aware that the food children eat influences not only their health but their behaviour. They are increasingly concerned about eating, but in a different way from previous generations. In the past, parents worried chiefly about *how much* children ate; now they are interested in *what* they eat. This book provides the newest, most detailed, specific, comprehensive, and authoritative information yet available on nutrition for children. Not only does it clear up parents' confusion about the best diet for their children but it also explains when and how to use nutritional supplements sensibly to give children's bodies the extra boost they need for maximum health. With increasing threats to their well-being from chemicals in the water, pesticides on fruits and vegetables, and other pollutants, children today need all the protection they can get. This unusual book will help you provide that protection.

Most mothers do try hard to feed their families correctly. But all too many are still playing by old rules. All too many have been incorrectly advised by their doctors: 'You don't need vitamins or food supplements. Just feed your child a balanced diet.'

Many paediatricians have received scant nutritional education themselves so they are not in a position to give parents the help they need and have a right to expect. In fact, readers will learn here that some elements of a so-called balanced diet can undermine the immune systems of their children.

The key to a healthy immune system is optimal nutrition. In this book, Dr Galland shows parents, step by step, what optimal nutrition is and how it interacts with their infants' or children's immune systems. It will be fascinating to the layperson to find out that a child's immune system has to *learn* to act effectively, and when it doesn't, it may respond to harmless or useful things as if they were enemies. When this happens, an allergy develops.

Dr Galland makes it very clear that a well-functioning immune system helps children not only to stay healthy and ward off allergies but also to heal themselves. Children do have a remarkable ability to heal themselves when they are properly nourished. Dr Galland explains how parents can remove nutritional impediments to optimal function so that children can heal as effectively as possible when illness strikes.

Many parents who have been working conscientiously to feed their families correctly will come to appreciate, while reading this book, that there is much more to it than they had realized. Dr Galland makes you aware that feeding yourself and your children adequately is not an easy thing to do. It is a very serious business and requires both knowledge and determination.

The scope of this volume is tremendous. Clear and specific advice about pregnancy is followed by invaluable recommendations about feeding infants, toddlers, school-age children, and teenagers to build up resistance.

Dr Galland also shows how nutrition affects children's behaviour. Child specialists gradually (and some reluctantly) are beginning to accept the fact that a child's behaviour as well as his or her health depends to a very great degree on the state of his or her body and how it is functioning. Even in the best and happiest of surroundings, children are not going to be able to function effectively unless they are properly nourished.

Books can be exciting for many different reasons. This one is exciting because, if its advice were followed, it could change the eating habits and improve the health of a whole generation of children. This is a book that I shall read and reread. It is a valuable addition to anybody's library and life.

I should like to conclude with Dr Galland's own closing statement: 'Optimal nutrition in childhood is a gift that lasts a lifetime.' Any parent who follows the instructions in this truly remarkable book will be in a position to give his or her child that priceless gift.

LOUISE BATES AMES
Associate Director and Co-Founder
Gesell Institute of Human Development

Preface

I have written this book in an attempt to meet the need for an up-to-date, practical and comprehensive guide for parents who want to raise very healthy children. Sound nutrition is the key to optimum immune function. Today, most parents recognize the truth of this notion but are confused about its implementation. The popular literature on nutrition suffers from several flaws: (1) much is outdated; (2) works from academic medical centres are confined to discussions of obesity and extreme malnutrition and are of little relevance to most parents; (3) the most sensational and publicized works have little scientific merit; and (4) ideas that may work well for adults are inappropriate for children. Infants, for example, fare very poorly on low-fat diets. Toddlers are usually intolerant of high-fibre diets. And pre-adolescents should generally not be given large doses of vitamins even though studies in adults show beneficial effects. The most important and widespread nutritional problems among Western children actually involve a deficiency of certain essential fats and the minerals required for their proper utilization in the body. This knowledge is only now beginning to extend from basic research into clinical medicine.

My interest in the science of nutrition extends back to my undergraduate studies at Harvard University 25 years ago. The biochemical pathways we studied were shown to be regulated by the presence of chemical co-factors. These co-factors were presented as if they were an intrinsic part of the body. In fact, we all knew that they were really nutrients – minerals and vitamins –

derived from food. It seemed to me then that nutrition determined bio-chemistry. During my training at Bellevue Hospital, I repeatedly witnessed the devastating effects of severe malnutrition on body chemistry and resist-ance to disease. Like most doctors, I could not relate those observations to patients who did not appear severely malnourished. When I began teaching family and community medicine and grappled with the problem of apparently normal people who did not respond as expected to medical treatment, I began to suspect that subtler forms of malnutrition might be the key. In fact, they were. My subsequent clinical research in this area substantiated my ideas and led to publications in scientific journals on the role of disturbances in fatty acid, magnesium and protein metabolism in chronic immune disorders.

When I joined the Gesell Institute of Human Development as director of medical research, I began applying to children the nutritional lessons I had learned in treating adults. I was impressed by the similarities and the differences created by age. Children respond much faster and much more completely to nutritional therapy than do adults. The younger the child, the faster the response. I found that most chronic illness among children can be treated or ameliorated by dietary measures. More important, I realized that most of the chronic health problems that plague young and middle-aged adults could have been prevented if those adults had been properly nourished as children. But children are not just small adults. At each stage of growth, they have special needs that must be met in specific ways. That understand-ing gave birth to this book.

Because the most critical deficiency among Western children is the dietary depletion of omega-3 essential fatty acids, Chapter 1 describes what these are, how they came to be depleted from our food, what the effects of this are, and what you, as a parent, can do about it. The key to raising children with healthy immune systems, and the core of this book, is understanding how to provide a proper supply of dietary omega-3 essential fatty acids and the co-factor minerals and vitamins your children need to utilize them fully.

Ideally, this process starts before birth, so Chapter 2 is devoted to optimal nutrition during pregnancy. In Chapter 3, I explain why human breast milk should be the only food your baby gets for his or her first six months of life, and how to keep your milk as healthy as it can be. If total or even partial breast-feeding is not possible, there are ways to overcome the inevitable deficits of bottle feeding, and these are outlined as well. Chapter 4 guides you through the introduction of various soft and solid foods to your child during the second six months of his or her life; it also surveys problems often encountered during that first year, such as feeding problems, colic, diar-rhoea, nappy rash and respiratory infections, and presents simple measures that I and others have found effective in correcting them.

Toddlers (ages 1 to 4) are the subject of Chapter 5, their quirks and special dietary needs. I have tried to emphasize the practical aspects of setting a lifelong pattern of sound nutrition that stresses these critical omega-3s and their mineral co-factors. Chapter 6 takes a look at the commonest toddler illnesses, such as ear infections, abdominal pain and allergies. Its goal is to give you the methods that I use in my medical practice to treat these problems nutritionally.

Chapter 7 follows your child to school, offering ideas on handling peer-group pressure to eat junk food. Healthy breakfasts, bag lunches and after-school snacks are presented and described. If your child has health or behavioural problems, there's more instruction on being a medical detective and using nutrition to help him or her get well.

Adolescence is the theme of Chapter 8. Now that your child's diet is largely beyond your control, here are ideas for motivating him or her and ensuring that most of his or her meals are healthy. The special needs of teenagers (different for boys and for girls) are explored. Nutritional approaches to acne, obesity, fatigue, colds, flu, headaches, glandular fever and optimum school performance are also presented.

In Chapter 9, I review the evidence that suggests that this programme will not only help you to raise robust and healthy youngsters, but will also help them resist the degenerative diseases of adulthood: cancer, coronary heart disease, high blood pressure, arthritis and other types of chronic inflammation.

In the recipes in Chapter 10, I've organized shopping hints and child-tested recipes for every meal plan in the text. There's special emphasis on creating nutritious snacks and desserts, because that's where your greatest challenge lies. The recipes were prepared with help from my family and from Carol Nostrand, author of *A Handbook for Improving Your Diet*.

This book is primarily designed to provide preventive health advice for parents. If your child is sick, you must consult your family doctor. If the recommendations in this book seem relevant to your child's illness, discuss them with the doctor, but do not attempt to make them a substitute for medical treatment.

I hope you will find in this book the spirit with which it was written. The most important nutrient of all is love. The nutritive superiority of human milk should be obvious to you when you read Chapter 3, but the joy of breast-feeding lies in the bonding between mother and baby. Feeding your family well is not easy. The pleasure in it comes from the love you share in taking care of each other.

DR LEO GALLAND

The Vital Link:
Nutrition and Your
Child's Immune System

Every mother wants healthy children. Good health should be a birthright, and no one is more aware of that than today's new parents. You belong to the most health-conscious generation in history. You want to raise robust children who can resist infection and disease, and who, because they are strong and healthy, will be able to use all their gifts of talent and intelligence to build successful lives.

In many ways, you are better equipped to do this than any parents have ever been. Yet, despite your best efforts, you may still, unwittingly, end up helping to weaken, rather than strengthen, your child's immune system. How? By serving foods that actually *prevent* infants and children from developing and maintaining the strong defences that nature has designed to protect them from disease.

Children have a remarkable ability to heal themselves; doctors and medication do not prevent or cure disease. When a child is given an antibiotic for an infection, you may think it is the antibiotic that cures the infection. It isn't. It is the child's immune system. The antibiotic just makes it a bit easier. If the immune system does not do its job, the antibiotic will be useless. When children are unable to cure themselves, chronic illness will result. In Western culture, there are a number of stumbling blocks to a well-functioning immune system that creates self-healing. Many of these are the result of nutritional mistakes. What those are, and what you, as a parent, can do about them is the subject of this book.

The key to a strong, healthy immune system is optimal nutrition. But what is good nutrition? The whole field of nutrition today is full of myths and mistaken ideas. Far too many nutritional consultants are operating on the basis of theories unsupported by scientific research. Paediatricians, the main source of feeding advice to parents, generally receive scant nutritional education themselves. And in any case, most of the principles we all learned in school are either incorrect or inappropriate in an era of ultra-processed and manufactured foods. Old ideas about a balanced diet (like the seven food groups, now the four food groups) cannot help you provide your child with optimal nutrition. In fact, some elements of a so-called balanced diet actually undermine the immune system. In addition, your children's bodies face new threats from chemicals in tap water and pesticide residues on fruits and vegetables. Environmental pollutants destroy or deplete their bodies' stores of many essential nutrients.

So, while medicine has conquered most of the traditional childhood diseases – diphtheria, measles, tetanus and polio – a host of new ills has arisen to plague today's children. Allergies are on the increase, and many children are bewilderingly prone to infections – recurrent ear infections are epidemic in wintertime. Immunologic diseases, Crohn's disease (a baffling inflammation of the intestines), multiple sclerosis and rheumatoid arthritis, all formerly rare, are on the rise among adolescents.

Fortunately, enough basic research has been done to master the *new* rules of the changed nutritional game. The past decade has yielded some major breakthroughs in our understanding of the relationship between nutrition and immunity. For most of that time, including three years at the Gesell Institute, the foremost child-development centre in the United States, I have been in the fortunate position of being a pioneer in the clinical application of this new nutritional research.

I have written this book to show parents exactly what optimal nutrition is and how it supports your children's immune systems – and your own, as well. You will learn how to lay a good foundation for your children's developing defences before they are born, and how to make sure that, during their crucial first year of life, their bodies build a top-notch protective shield. Then I will take you, step by step, through all the phases of your children's development and show you how, at each stage, you can help them to safeguard and maintain their bodies' defences so that they, in turn, can help them mature into healthy, vigorous adults.

The immune system is made up of an army of special cells ready to go into action at a moment's notice. Immune cells attack and destroy anything foreign that invades the body or threatens it from within – from bacteria and viruses to cancers. A healthy immune system is always on the alert, its cells patrolling the body to nip tumours in the bud, zap the bacteria that swarm in when your children cut their fingers, and fight the viruses that give them colds and flu.

Whatever your children's ages, you can apply optimal nutrition to enhance their resistance to disease, starting right now. Past mistakes *can* be remedied. It is *never* too late to help your children improve their immunity.

ESSENTIAL FATTY ACIDS: THE SPECIAL NUTRIENTS YOUR CHILDREN'S IMMUNE SYSTEMS NEED

My own research and clinical work, and the work of many other researchers and clinicians, suggests that the key to a healthy immune system is found in substances called *essential fatty acids*, or EFAs. You may already have read or seen on television the news that EFAs can reduce cholesterol and protect against heart disease. You may even know that fatty, cold-water fish and fish oil are a rich source of EFAs. But very few people yet realize that EFAs are crucial to the health of their own and their children's immune systems.

EFAs are essential because:

● Your children need them to maintain health – especially to maintain their immune systems.
● Your children's bodies can't make them. They must come from the food they eat.

And that's where the problem starts. Our eating patterns have changed radically over the last 100 years – so much so that, today, we are in the midst of a famine. It's not the kind of famine that has, historically, decimated the immunity of whole nations. That kind of famine is easy to understand: it produces starvation and a critical lack of protein for use by the body.

The famine we face today is more subtle, a product of highly developed, mainly Western culture. It's hard to believe, because our supermarkets are packed with fresh produce and boxes and cans of everything, but we are literally starving for essential fatty acids or EFAs.

EFAs are found in many foods, but they are most richly concentrated in the oils of certain nuts, seed and fish. Nuts, seeds and beans aren't important items in the diets of most of us. Partly because of this, and partly because we eat much less fish than we used to – and overprocess most of what we do eat – one whole group of EFAs has been virtually eliminated from our diets.

Even those of us who are careful to use vegetable oils for cooking aren't necessarily getting the EFAs we need. EFAs are fragile, easily damaged by air, high temperatures and food processing. Most of the oil we consume today has been heavily processed.

What's more, your children's need for EFAs depends to a great extent on other factors in their diet. If they eat a lot of the wrong kinds of fats, or don't get enough of certain essential vitamins and minerals, for example, their bodies may not be able to make proper use of the EFAs they consume. For all these reasons, we are in the midst of an epidemic of EFA deficiencies that is undermining the health of our children. That's the bad news. The good news is that you as parents can resolve this crisis in your children. You will need to follow some clear, simple guidelines offered in the pages that follow.

WHAT ARE EFAs AND WHERE CAN YOU FIND THEM?

Most of you know that there are good and bad fats. All the media, from your morning newspaper to your evening TV news, have been telling you for years to cut down on saturated fats and eat more unsaturated fats. Saturated fats, they warn you, will clog your arteries, raise your cholesterol level and, ultimately, cause a heart attack. So you sauté or stir-fry with vegetable oil and serve margarine or one of the new spreads instead of butter. Even some fast-food outlets have switched from beef tallow to partially hydrogenated vegetable oils for deep-frying their chicken nuggets and fish fillets. This is all part of a healthy trend, right?

Wrong. To understand how the right kinds of fats can not only bolster your children's immune systems but can also reverse some of the damage done by the wrong kinds of fats, you need to know more about how fats work.

Fatty acids are the chemical building blocks of fat, and they come in two varieties: saturated and unsaturated. Saturated fatty acids make a fat that is stiff and solid at room temperature, such as beef fat and hard cheese. Your bodies need some saturated fatty acids, but they aren't essential – *your children's bodies can make all they need.* All the saturated fatty acids they consume are completely unnecessary. Not only do they clog up the arteries but they can also interfere with the body's ability to use EFAs.

Unsaturated fatty acids make a fat that is liquid at room temperature. They comprise most vegetable oils: corn, safflower, peanut, soya, olive and others. Essential fatty acids are all unsaturated, but – here's the catch – *not all unsaturated fatty acids are essential.* And, as with saturated fats, your children's bodies can make all the non-essential unsaturated fatty acids they need out of other foods. What's more, if they eat a lot of non-essential fatty acids, these can interfere even more than saturated fatty acids with the body's ability to use EFAs.

Unfortunately, most of the vegetable oils that we consume are loaded with non-essential fatty acids, many of which are created in a manufacturing process called *hydrogenation.* In order to prolong shelf life, hydrogenation converts unsaturated fats into saturated fats. If you read labels, you know how hard it is to find any food in a can or package that does not list 'hydrogenated vegetable oil' or, even more often, 'partially hydrogenated vegetable oil' as an ingredient. Partial hydrogenation is actually worse, because it physically alters any EFAs in the oil to create *artificial* unsaturated fatty acids. These artificial fatty acids are not only unnatural and unnecessary, they can also have a disastrous effect on the ability of your children's bodies to use EFAs.

Soya oil, a perfectly good oil that, when unprocessed, contains useful amounts of EFAs, is usually consumed as a partially hydrogenated ingredient of manufactured foods, from biscuits to spaghetti sauce. Palm oil, also frequently used in processed foods, contains saturated – that is, non-essential – fatty acids even in its natural state. It needs no hydrogenation to be harmful.

Olive oil's fatty acids are non-essential in its natural state, but it can be a good cooking oil none the less. It is stable, so it doesn't break down during storage or cooking to form substances that harm EFAs. It has also been shown to lower blood cholesterol levels.

The EFA Families

There are two kinds, or families, of EFAs. The *omega-6* family is found mainly in seeds grown in temperate climates – safflower, sunflower and corn oils are all rich in omega-6 EFAs. It is also found in evening primrose oil. Because of the long-term trend towards using vegetable oils in cooking and salad dressings, most children today get plenty of omega-6 oils – but, as we shall see, many have problems in using them.

The EFA famine among Western children mainly involves the other family: *omega-3* EFAs. Only one vegetable oil is really rich in omega-3s: food-grade linseed oil (also known as flaxseed oil). Soyabean, walnut and wheat-germ oils may also contain significant amounts of omega-3s if their source plants were grown in a cold climate and if they are fresh, cold-pressed* and not hydrogenated. Freshly ground wheat germ is a good source, too, but it is hard to get and spoils rapidly.

* An important note about oil processing: no oil is truly cold-pressed. The act of pressing generates heat; the harder or drier the seed, the more pressure needed and the more heat generated. Most commercial oils are extracted with extra heat added to enhance the extraction process. This can create high temperatures, which damage the EFAs. The best oils are those extracted without added heat ('cold-pressed'). After extraction, the oil must be clarified. Unrefined oils are clarified by centrifugation and filtration. They tend to be dark and have distinctive flavours. Refined oils are extracted into hexane (petrol). The fatty acids dissolve in the hexane, which is then boiled off. Most commercial oils are solvent-extracted with hexane to produce greater clarity, a lighter colour and a blander taste. Because solvent extraction removes some trace minerals, it also prolongs shelf life. Solvent extraction has little effect on the EFA content of an oil, however. Many food oils are then bleached, to further lighten colour. This destroys some EFAs and naturally occurring anti-oxidants (*see below*, p. 10) such as vitamin E. Partial hydrogenation is the final step in destroying their nutritional value, as it converts EFAs into artificial, non-essential fatty acids. The oils you buy should never be bleached or hydrogenated; they should be pressed without added heat; and, if possible, they should be unrefined as well.

The other important sources of omega-3 EFAs are cod-liver oil and fresh fish – oily, cold-water fish such as salmon, tuna, mackerel, herring and sardines. The key word here is *fresh*. Canning causes some loss of EFAs, especially if vegetable oil is added.

Both processing and cooking can destroy the EFAs in fish. In addition, many kinds of popular seafood – sole and flounder are good examples – aren't rich enough in EFAs to be good sources in the first place. The breaded and fried or deep-fried fillets of fish served by so many restaurants and fish and chip chops, and sold frozen in all supermarkets, contain few EFAs to start with. Worse, this method of preparation is often accomplished with the aid of partially hydrogenated vegetable oils. And frying or deep-frying, as we shall see later in this chapter, produces chemicals that harm EFAs.

There is one good, inexpensive source of both omega-6 and omega-3 EFAs: dried beans, such as kidney and haricot beans, and soya beans. A family that eats these beans regularly can meet all its EFA needs.

The foods that supply EFAs are actually the goods our bodies were designed to eat. Early humans were hunters and gatherers. Most of the fat they ate came from seeds, nuts, game and fish. Game is very low in fat but rich in EFAs, including omega-3 EFAs. People living near the sea have always consumed lots of fish.

Linseed oil was a staple food oil all over northern Europe, from Scandinavia east to Siberia, right up to World War II. And a century ago, many people were still eating a lot of cold-water fish. At one point, British labourers demanded that their employers not serve salmon for lunch more than four times a week. But overfishing has made many EFA-containing fish too expensive for regular fare today.

Without knowing anything about EFAs, your grandparents knew that cod-liver oil, a rich source of omega-3s, was a good thing to give children in the winter. Cold increases the body's need for EFAs. While they were giving it for vitamins A and D, they were also supplying a cold-weather EFA boost.

The past 50 years have been disastrous for EFAs in our diets. As traditional sources of omega-3s disappeared, industrial countries learned to hydrogenate oils, destroying the omega-3s they contained. The hydrogenization of vegetable oils has also added large quantities of non-essential fats to our diets. Fish processors fillet the fish, discard the EFA-rich organs, and replace the oil with water. And we have added large quantities of sugar to our children's diets, interfering even more with their bodies' abilities to use EFAs.

At the same time, our children's bodies are increasingly deficient in certain minerals and vitamins that are necessary to help them process and use EFAs. And the ever-growing numbers of chemical pollutants in our food, water and air, together with such pervasive cooking methods as deep-frying, are promoting the destruction of the EFAs in our children's bodies.

To understand how these different factors have brought us to the brink of an EFA disaster – and to understand how you can pull your children out of it – you need to know something about how their bodies use EFAs.

THE PROSTAGLANDIN CONNECTION

In each of the two main families of essential fatty acids, there is one particularly important acid: In the omega-6 family, it is *linoleic acid*, or LA. In the omega-3 family, it is *linolenic acid*, or LNA. But neither of these acids is, by itself, of any use to your children's bodies – both must be converted into other chemical forms. The body does this through the series of chemical reactions, regulated by different enzymes, that is called metabolism.

To do their job of regulating EFA metabolism properly, enzymes depend on the presence of certain key *co-factor* vitamins (B_6, A, C and E) and minerals (magnesium, zinc, copper and selenium). If your children get a good supply of all these vitamins and minerals, their bodies will metabolize LA and LNA into a special group of hormone-like substances called *prostaglandins*. Among other things, prostaglandins seem to regulate the activity of the white blood cells in the immune system, for instance, the *T-cells* and *B-cells*, which are the major classes of *lymphocytes*.

These cells are divided, rather like an army, into specialists with different areas of responsibility. *Macrophages* patrol the bloodstream looking for both microbial invaders and debris, which they clean up. (*Macrophage* means literally 'large eaters'.) If a macrophage does encounter a bacterium, it takes an antigen molecule from it and carries it around until it meets a helper *T-cell*.

The cells that give the orders are the T-cells: *helper T-cells* send the *killer T-cells* and the *B-cells* into action. B-cells, once prodded into action by the helper T-cells, produce *antibodies*, while *suppressor T-cells* issue ceasefire orders when the battle is won.

B-cells and T-cells are the mind of the immune system, and they are unique. They are the only cells in the body, besides brain cells, that have memory. *Lymphocytes learn and remember who is a friend and who is an enemy.*

An infant's and small children's immune system may have marshalled its army, but, as I pointed out earlier, it is an ignorant army. It has not yet been challenged. It knows who its friends are – the body it inhabits, the foods that come into that body, and the good bacteria that help the body work. But it is meeting enemies for the first time. For each new enemy, it must figure out the right antibody and the right response for its disease-fighting cells. That's where the lymphocytes come in. B-cells learn how to make antibodies for every one of the thousands of different germs, toxins, fungi, bacteria, viruses and parasites that invade the body in the course of a lifetime. T-cells remember every invader so that, each time they come across it, they can instantly order out the troops. A specific germ may make some headway the first time, but the second time it invades, the army will be ready.

The immune system's army works as a team, and, like any other team, it depends on a constant exchange of information, or signals, among its members. The T-cells are the key to that communication. Their state of health is critical, because they make decisions and give orders. Their ability to do that may depend, in turn, on the right supplies of prostaglandins. Experiments with animals have shown that, when prostaglandin production goes awry, it is the T-cells that are the most disastrously affected. And when they can't do their jobs, the whole immune system malfunctions.

If something goes wrong with their bodies' production of prostaglandins, then – if not enough of one or too much of another is made – your children's defences may well be crippled. The result may be disease.

Your children's bodies make 50 different prostaglandins. Problems in their production can be detected behind a host of 20th-century illnesses, including cancer, asthma and other allergies, and auto-immune diseases such as lupus and rheumatoid arthritis.

When treating children with what I suspect might be a prostaglandin imbalance, the first thing I look for is whether they are getting enough EFAs. But suppose they are eating plenty of foods that contain both LA (linoleic acid) and LNA (linolenic acid)? The next culprit I look for is a deficiency in the key co-factor vitamins and minerals that make it possible for enzymes to regulate the metabolism of LA and LNA. These, you will recall, are vitamins B_6, A, C and E, and the minerals magnesium, zinc, copper and selenium. If children's diets are deficient in even one of these co-factor nutrients, this will have the same effect as an EFA deficiency. In my medical practice, I see this over and over.

It is no accident that the foods that are naturally rich in EFAs are also naturally rich in the EFA co-factor nutrients. Nuts, seeds and beans are excellent sources of magnesium, copper, zinc and vitamins E and B_6. Seafood is a rich source of all the minerals. If fresh vegetables are added for vitamins A and C, we have a balanced, EFA-strong diet that can't be bettered for its immune-building effect.

Unfortunately, children today get most of their calories from sugar, processed cereal grains such as wheat and maize, processed oils, dairy products and fatty meats. It's no wonder that most children today consume far too little magnesium, vitamin B_6 and copper – in fact, in the United States they consume less than two-thirds of the US Recommended Dietary Allowance (US RDA).

Zinc and vitamin A deficiencies are very common, too. A zinc deficiency is most likely to occur in young children who get most of their nutrients from milk and cheese. Vitamin A deficiencies most often show up in adolescents who live on meat, potatoes and fast foods, and who shun vegetables and eggs.

If children's diets are rich in sources of both EFAs and the co-factor nutrients but they still show signs of an EFA deficiency, then the culprit will almost always be *anti-nutrients*, the bane of every nutrition-conscious parent. Anti-nutrients are foods or substances that not only have little or no nutritional value but also block or make EFA metabolism go awry. The list of these villains in the Westen diet is far too long:

● *Non-essential Fatty Acids.* Major anti-nutrients, they confuse the enzymes that regulate EFA metabolism into metabolizing them instead of the EFAs. Topping the whole list are partially hydrogenated vegetable oils, which interfere with the enzyme action. Unlike sugar, which fills what some scientists think may be a biological need for sweetness, these artificial fats fill no human need.

● *Sugar.* Large quantities weaken the enzymes of EFA metabolism. Sugar supplies a relatively huge proportion of the calories consumed by most children, but brings with it none of the vitamins and minerals needed for EFA metabolism or for energy. If children eat wholewheat bread, they get with it the B vitamins and magnesium needed both to convert the bread into energy and as co-factor nutrients. These are naturally present in wholewheat flour. But if they eat sweets, or white-flour pastries, they have to get those B vitamins and minerals from some other food.

Recent studies in both animals and humans have shown that sugar increases the adverse effects of a copper deficiency, although the mechanism by which it does so hasn't been discovered yet. Sugar also increases the amounts of magnesium and other important minerals that are excreted in the urine.[1]*

● *Sodium.* Common salt – sodium chloride – is naturally present in many foods. The amount found in unprocessed foods is enough for children living in temperate or cold climates. But large amounts of salt are used in processing foods: many researchers think that the salt intake of those of us in the West is *10 to 20 times* that necessary to maintain sodium balance in the body. This not only contributes to the development of high blood pressure, it also increases the amounts of magnesium (a co-factor nutrient) and potassium that are lost in the urine. This constant depletion means that children have to get much more of these two key minerals in their food or in supplements.

* References appear at the end of this book.

● *Phosphates.* Phosphorus, like sodium, is an essential mineral, but, also like sodium, children get far too much of it. Phosphates are used as preservatives in many foods, and phosphoric acid is used to keep fizzy drinks bubbly. Meat is naturally rich in phosphates. Large amounts of phosphorus in the system act as a kind of intestinal sludge, blocking the absorption of calcium and magnesium, both of which are important for many other reasons besides their crucial roles as co-factor nutrients in EFA metabolism.

● *Pesticides.* These are sprayed on fruits, vegetables and grains to kill insects and fungi, and their residues remain in or on these foods when you eat them. Some herbicides that contaminate agricultural produce interfere with the body's ability to use vitamin B_6, which means that more of this co-factor vitamin must be provided in foods or supplements.[2] Vitamin B_6 deficiency not only interferes with EFA metabolism, but it may also have neurological effects ranging from epileptic seizures to a feeling of pins and needles in the hands.

● *Free radicals.* Your child's cells use oxygen to burn food for energy and to burn away germs and foreign chemicals such as pesticides. This process of combustion creates tiny bonfires in the cells, and these fires give off 'sparks' that can start fires in undesirable places, damaging cell membranes and destroying EFAs. The chemical name for these sparks is *free radicals*.

Frying foods in oil creates free radicals when high heat damages the oil. Fast-food restaurants keep cooking oil bubbling all day to deep-fry chips, fish and chicken, worsening the damage by the hour. Your children eat the free radicals with their chips and chicken nuggets, and the heat-damaged oils create more free radicals in their bodies.

Fortunately, the body has a 'fire brigade' to snuff these sparks before they start too many fires. This band of free-radical quenchers is called the *anti-oxidant defence system*. The anti-oxidant defence system depends for its effectiveness on a number of vitamins and minerals, particularly vitamins A, C, E, B_2 (riboflavin) and B_3 (nicotinic acid) and the minerals zinc, copper, manganese and sulphur. Exposure to environmental pollutants such as pesticides in foods increases your children's need for these anti-oxidants, especially for vitamins C and E, both of which are destroyed in the firefighting process.[3]

Anti-oxidants are crucial to a child's immune system, too. When white blood cells kill germs, they generate relatively enormous amounts of heat, turning into tiny furnaces. They need a generous supply of anti-oxidants to keep them from literally burning themselves up within the body.

So your children need anti-oxidants to protect both their EFAs and the individual cells of their immune systems. Heat-damaged oils and pollutants in food and the environment dramatically increase their need for these key vitamins and minerals.

HOW THE IMMUNE SYSTEM CAN MALFUNCTION

The unborn infant's developing immune system is learning how to recognize 'me' – the infant's own body and everything that belongs in it. A perfectly functioning immune system learns and remembers that it should not attack anything that is 'me'. Once it learns that, it can concentrate its energies on attacking everything that is 'not me'.

But sometimes something goes wrong, and a person's immune system responds to harmless or useful things as if they were enemies; it reacts, say, to a piece of bread as if it were a virus, or responds to the body's own thyroid gland as if it were a cancer. When the immune system attacks harmless or even useful things that enter the body from outside, whether food or plant spores, we call it an *allergy*. When the immune system attacks the body it inhabits, an *auto-immune disease* develops.

In my practice, I see many children with allergic illnesses, and in most cases, EFA deficiency plays an important role. Jason's story is one dramatic example.

At 12, Jason had many food and pollen allergies. He was also hyperactive and displayed two signals of EFA deficiency: he was always thirsty and his skin was very dry. I enriched Jason's diet with safflower oil, a polyunsaturated oil rich in EFAs, and cut down on the amount of sugar he consumed. Almost immediately, he became less thirsty and his skin soon became soft and shiny. More important, he calmed down and his food allergies disappeared.

The LA in the safflower oil allowed Jason to increase his output of *prostaglandin E_1*, or PGE_1. PGE_1 is a natural suppressor of allergic reactions and a hormonal regulator of the nervous system; so, in addition to curing Jay's allergies, it cured his hyperactivity. (Many prostaglandins do two or more jobs; thus when you bolster your children's immune systems, you are also contributing to the healthy regulation of their nervous systems, their hearts and blood vessels and their glandular systems.)

My research shows that people who have allergies need more EFAs than people who don't.[4] The reason seems to be that, in people with allergies, one of the enzymes involved in EFA metabolism is weakened or doesn't function properly. Drs David Horrobin and Mehar Manku of the Efamol Research Institute in Nova Scotia, Canada have found that, in children with allergic eczema (dermatitis) and asthma, the first step in making PGE_1 – the conversion of LA to an intermediate fatty acid known as GLA – is blocked.[5] Dr Ross Rocklin of Tufts University in Massachusetts has found a similar block in people with simple hay fever.[6]

Although the weakness of this enzyme is undoubtedly inherited, the condition is made worse by a deficiency of EFAs. The good news is that it can be overcome by adding enough EFAs to the diet.

We shall explore the question of allergies in more detail in Chapters 6 and 9. Here, I want to point out that *even when an infant inherits a predisposition for allergies, special protective elements found in breast milk, together with EFAs, can delay the onset of allergic illness and greatly reduce its severity.*

As I will discuss throughout this book, proper EFA intake is also helpful to children who suffer from recurrent infections, which frequently go along with allergies.

Auto-immune diseases aren't common in young children, but they are appearing with increasing frequency in adolescents. Diabetes, Crohn's disease, ulcerative colitis, systemic lupus and juvenile rheumatoid arthritis are, sadly, striking more and more young people between the ages of 12 and 21. In many cases, it appears that unbalanced prostaglandin synthesis, in which certain harmful prostaglandins are produced in excess, plays an important role in the development of the illness.

Feeding fish oils to experimental animals has been shown to prevent the development of auto-immune diseases similar to lupus, multiple sclerosis and rheumatoid arthritis. I find EFA supplements empirically useful in treating children with established auto-immune disorders.

THE SIGNS OF EFA DEFICIENCY

In addition to their crucial role in regulating the immune system, EFAs are a vital component of all your body's membranes – from the membrane around each cell, which allows it to function properly, to your skin, the body's outer membrane. Because your skin's outermost layer is composed of cell membranes and protein, an EFA deficiency produces dry, scaly skin.

A healthy child has lustrous skin, and hair that reflects light without the aid of conditioners and oils. (Hair is really an appendage of the skin. It is made of protein derived from cell membrane, and its condition closely reflects that of the skin.) Few children have such hair and skin today. Instead, varying degrees of dryness are the rule – from a flat dullness (referred to as a 'matt finish' by Sid Baker of the Gesell Institute) to visible scaling and roughness.

There is an easy way to tell whether your children's dry skin is caused by an EFA deficiency: increase their omega-3 intake by following the guidelines in this book. The chances are that their hair and skin will soon acquire their own lustre. (If you have the same problems, or if your nails are brittle or you sometimes get tiny lumps, like a rash, on the backs of your arms, you can try the same test on yourself.)

Most experts agree that this kind of *functional test* – in which you give increasing doses of a particular nutrient to see how a specific condition changes – is the only accurate way to assess a person's nutritional status. It is the basis for my own and other specialists' work with nutritionally deficient patients.

HOW TO MAKE SURE YOUR CHILDREN GET ENOUGH EFAs

Throughout this book, there will be guidelines to help you make sure your children get the EFAs they need. The key is a balanced intake of fatty acids, and the best way to do this is through food.

As we have shown, good dietary sources of EFAs are nuts, seeds, beans and some types of fish. EFA requirements vary somewhat with climate. To maintain a relationship between omega-3s and omega-6s suitable for most people living in the United Kingdom, the best nuts are home-produced walnuts, the best seed is food-quality linseed and the best beans are haricot, kidney and soya. The best fish are fresh salmon, tuna, mackerel, bluefish, sardines or herring.

But it is clearly not practical to expect you to ensure that your children get three servings each week of fresh salmon or tuna, plus plenty of walnuts, flaxseed and beans. For the vast majority of parents, food oils are the best and most practical way to suply EFAs to their children.

● *Linseed oil.* For most children, the best oil is food-grade linseed oil. It contains a mixture of omega-3s and omega-6s, with the 3s predominating. I prefer it because the EFAs that it contains are in a form that gives a child's body better control over EFA metabolism than do those in other oils, and because of its bland taste.

The antipodean firm, Blackmores Laboratories Ltd, has begun marketing cold-pressed food-grade linseed oil in this country. This is a superior product, unrefined and labelled with a 'use by' date. It will keep for up to two months in the refrigerator. It can also be kept frozen – it won't solidify because it is pure polyunsaturated fat – for four months. If your local healthfood shop doesn't stock it, they will usually be happy to order it for you.

Freshly pressed linseed oil is slightly sweet. Usually, the linseed oil you buy will have almost no taste. *If it tastes even slightly bitter, it is rancid; throw it out.*

(Under no circumstances buy the linseed oil that is used by artists and decorators; it is poisonous.)

Some people, even quite young children, have no difficulty swallowing a tablespoon of linseed oil right before eating or before drinking a glass of juice. If there is any problem with this, you can stir linseed oil into orange juice (stir vigorously and drink immediately – the oil forms a suspension and will separate out quickly).

You can use linseed oil as a dressing on hot vegetables or pasta or in salad dressing. For flavour, mix equal amounts of linseed oil and olive oil. Other salad dressings you can make are mayonnaise made with linseed oil, and linseed oil blended with yogurt or soft tofu and flavoured with herbs.

For some spreads, mix equal amounts of linseed oil and butter – this is better than all the substitute spreads on the market, including margarine. (Margarine is made of partially hydrogenated vegetable oil, an arch anti-nutrient.) Linseed oil can also be mixed with yoghurt and flavoured with sugar-free jam or pear and apple spread.

Finally, you can add a tablespoon of linseed oil to a health shake (see Chapter 10).

Don't use linseed oil for frying or sautéing, since high heat plus oxygen destroys its EFAs. It can, however, be used in baking, because EFAs aren't destroyed in this kind of cooking process (see Chapter 10).

Linseed oil is absorbed through the skin, and I sometimes recommend rubbing it on the skin of infants, but it smells slightly fishy.

Linseed oil is the very best source of EFA omega-3s. If it is unavailable, you can substitute 2 tablespoons (30 ml) of walnut oil for 1 tablespoon (15 ml) of linseed oil. Unfortunately, walnut oil is expensive. You may also substitute 1 teaspoon (5 ml) of cod-liver oil for 1 tablespoon (15 ml) of linseed oil.

● *Cod-liver oil.* A fine source of omega-3s and vitamins A and D, but these vitamins can be toxic in large amounts. Because of this, I never administer more than 1 teaspoon (5 ml) of cod-liver oil a day to young children, or 1 tablespoon (15 ml) to adolescents. Taste is a problem, even when the cod-liver oil is mixed into juice. Flavoured cod-liver oil is available, and you may find this more palatable. Never use defatted cod-liver oil. Taking the fat out makes cod-liver oil taste better, but it also removes its nutrient value.

● *Fish-oil extracts.* These are marketed in capsules under brand names such as MaxEPA, which can be found at healthfood shops. The safe dosage is 2–8 capsules a day, the lowest dosage being given to children. If children are too young to swallow the capsules, the capsules can be cut and the oil rubbed into the thin skin of the inner forearm or thigh, from where it will be well absorbed.

I find fish-oil extracts useful in treating diseases associated with EFA deficiency, but I don't recommend them for preventive purposes. If your children's dry skin does not become supple with a combination of the diet I recommend and some linseed oil, a month-long trial of fish-oil supplementation will establish whether they need omega-3 EFAs in the form in which the latter occur in fish. *Warning: those with blood disorders or bleeding problems should only take fish-oil extracts under medical supervision.*

• *Evening primrose oil and blackcurrant seed oil.* Some children, like Jason, whose story I told earlier, need a higher intake of omega-6 EFAs than a balanced diet will supply. This is especially true of hyperactive children, those with allergies, and children who seem to be thirsty all the time. If your children's skin remains dry despite a healthy diet, linseed oil and fish oils, then they may have an increased need for omega-6s.

One or two tablespoons (15–30 ml) of safflower oil a day may be useful, but more efficient, and more expensive, sources of omega-6s are evening primrose and blackcurrant seed oils. These seed oils are unique in containing GLA (gamma-linolenic acid), a fatty acid produced as an intermediate step during the metabolism of linoleic acid (LA). GLA enables a child's body to bypass the most common block in omega-6 metabolism.

A reliable source of GLA is Efamol (brand) evening primrose oil, available from healthfood shops. Evening primrose oil comes in 250- or 500-milligram (mg) capsules, which can be swallowed by an older child or cut open for the oil to be rubbed on an infant's or small child's skin, through which it is slowly absorbed into the body. Dosage varies from 1 to 4 g a day; the smallest dose (four 250-mg capsules or two 500-mg capsules) should be given to children. *Warning: those with any form of epilepsy should not take evening primrose oil except under medical supervision.*

Since real primrose oil is expensive, a number of products claiming to offer GLA at a reduced price have appeared on the market. Some call themselves primrose oil, but, in fact, are mostly soya oil. Avoid them. Blackcurrant seed oil has recently emerged as a source of GLA, too. One 250-mg capsule is equivalent in GLA to one 500-mg capsule of evening primrose oil. One brand of blackcurrant seed oil is Glanolin, produced by GR Lane Health Products Ltd and available from healthfood shops.

Food oils in the United States

Fish oils have proved effective in treating a large number of diseases in animal experiments and clinical trials, and have shown virtually no toxicity and a minimum of side-effects. In humans, they help to lower cholesterol, triglycerides and blood pressure; decrease complications of diabetes; and improve arthritis, psoriasis, asthma, colitis and migraines. In animals, they help to prevent heart attacks, cancer and auto-immune diseases. No drug or nutritional supplement has a comparable record of efficacy and safety in scientific studies. If you understand the widespread role of prostaglandins in disease and the effect of diet on prostaglandin formation, this record will not surprise you. In the United States, manufacturers of fish-oil concentrates have used this research to promote their products commercially, and the Food and Drug Administration, the US government watchdog, has taken umbrage, asserting that such advertising makes fish-oil extracts drugs, not food supplements.

Evening primrose oil has shown more limited and inconsistent benefits in experimental and clinical studies, but some of its US distributors have been even more vociferous in asserting its value in the treatment and prevention of illness. The FDA has recently banned the importing of primrose oil into the US for that reason.

In an even more foolish and dangerous decision, the FDA has moved to limit the availability of linseed oil to American consumers, claiming that its safety as a food oil has not been proved. At the same time, there is *no restriction* on the use or sale of hydrogenated vegetable oils, even though numerous studies in animals have shown that the artificial fatty acids they contain may have toxic and undesirable effects. Hydrogenated oils have been in use for a mere 50 years, whereas linseed oil has been a tradition in Northern and Central Europe for centuries and flax meal has been used for millennia. The safety of linseed oil is documented and established by a long tradition of use. Alternatives to linseed oil include cod-liver and walnut oils and unhydrogenated oils extracted from northern soya beans and winter wheat. The FDA's attempts to deny to American consumers access to linseed oil is such a serious disservice to the people of that country that it warrants an investigation of the agency and the origins of that decision.

In the chapters that follow, I will outline for you how, during each stage of your children's lives, from conception to young adulthood, you can help them build resistance to disease through an optimum intake of EFAs, their co-factor nutrients and anti-oxidants, and by avoiding anti-nutrients. This book will resolve any confusion you may have about the best diet for your children, and it will give you the advice you need to use nutritional supplements rationally and sensibly to give your children's bodies the extra boost they need for maximum health. There is no magic here – just the foods and supplements that have been proved effective by research and in my own medical practice.

Pregnancy:
Optimally Nourished Mothers
Produce Stronger Babies

2

Your unborn child's future lies in your hands. From conception to birth, he will be completely dependent on you for the nourishment that will largely determine whether he is born healthy. A developing foetus gets all his nourishment from the placenta, which, in turn, is kept supplied by his mother's blood. So *everything* you take in – food, drinks, drugs, cigarette smoke – will affect your baby's development. Moreover, he will depend on your immune system to protect him from germs that attack you. Since everything you ingest also affects the condition of your own body's defences, it is very important for you to get enough minerals, vitamins and EFAs, and to eat and drink as few anti-nutrients as possible.

The choices – what you eat, whether or not you smoke, whether you drink alcohol, what drugs you take – are all yours. If the child you are carrying is born with the healthiest possible body, he will have the foundation for a well-regulated defence system that will grow stronger as he grows older. Of course, you can start later in your child's life to counteract earlier nutritional mistakes, but why not start him off right?

The first three months of pregnancy (i.e. the first trimester) are the most dangerous in terms of birth defect, because the cells of the embryo and foetus are multiplying and specializing very rapidly.

During the second and third trimesters, the foetus grows into a fully formed baby. This is when his immune cells develop, but they aren't yet able to do any work. Your own immune system does all the work for both of you.

Not until three months after birth will your infant's immune system begin to protect him.

We know little about how the foods a mother eats specifically affect her unborn baby's immune system, but a great deal is known about the ways in which what you eat and drink affect his overall development. So it's a safe bet that good nutrition will help his immune system to develop properly.

The first rule of good nutrition for a pregnant woman is one that will make food lovers happy: *Eat heartily.* Since your primary goal is to ensure good nutrition for your unborn baby, quantity, as well as quality, is important. *Do not skip meals, skimp on food or attempt to diet during your pregnancy.*

This means that, as long as you are eating nutritionally balanced meals, limiting the amount of weight you gain should never be a goal during pregnancy. If you start with a normal weight – not more than 20 pounds over what you should weigh for your height and bone structure – you must gain 25 to 35 pounds over nine months. Even if you are more than 20 pounds overweight at the beginning of your pregnancy, you must still gain between 24 to 27 pounds. Unborn babies have first call on all their mothers' nutrients; if there isn't enough for two, the mothers' bodies will go without – hardly the best way to begin life with a new baby. Of course, if any essential nutrients are lacking or in very low quantities, both mother and baby will suffer.

The weight you gain represents your baby, the placenta, the amniotic fluid, and your expanded breasts and blood volume. Any excess weight you carry before pregnancy is mainly fat, which will do your unborn baby little good. He will need protein, calcium and all the other crucial minerals and vitamins. (If you are not sure whether your prepregnancy weight is normal, check the most recent height/weight tables issued by many insurance companies. Many women feel they are overweight when their weight is, in fact, normal, and feel normal only when they are quite thin. The tables should set you straight.)

What if you find that you gain a lot of weight very quickly – if, say, in the first three-to-six months you put on all the weight you expected to gain over the entire nine-month period? The same advice still holds: don't diet. It is far less dangerous to your baby's health for you to continue to gain weight (although you should bring your weight gain to the attention of the doctor or midwife at your antenatal clinic). Once your baby is born, you can safely begin reducing your food intake. The larger your weight gain, the longer it will take to lose it. (But if you breast-feed, you will need to keep on eating for two until your baby is weaned.)

Are three meals a day enough? Probably not. During pregnancy, you will feel your best if you change your eating pattern to six small, low-fat, high-carbohydrate meals. Why? There are two reasons:

• Many such mini-meals will help keep you from overeating, because you will be less likely to want between-meal snacks.

- You may avoid three of the commonest conditions of pregnancy: *nausea*, *hypoglycaemia*, and *hyperglycaemia*.

Nausea

Also known as morning sickness, this is not an inevitable accompaniment to the earliest stages of pregnancy. When severe, it may actually be caused by nutritional deficiencies. A six-mini-meal-a-day pattern will often relieve it. (For more information on nausea, *see* p. 37.)

Hypoglycaemia

This is a condition in which the amount of sugar (glucose) in the blood falls so low that not enough gets to the brain; it is often the culprit when a pregnant woman faints. Hypoglycaemia can also create hormonal swings that make you feel listless and down in the dumps. But, most crucial of all, *when your blood sugar is low, your developing infant's blood sugar is low, too – and lack of sufficient glucose can damage an unborn baby's brain*. So you want to avoid hypoglycaemia.

Hyperglycaemia

High blood sugar is technically the opposite of hypoglycaemia. In fact, the two often accompany each other. The hormonal changes of pregnancy can produce wide swings in blood sugar levels, with hyperglycaemia being followed by hypoglycaemia. Severe hyperglycaemia is a sign of diabetes, a dangerous condition in pregnancy. A recent study from Italy, published in the *New England Journal of Medicine*, found that even the mildest degrees of hyperglycaemia in pregnancy, generally considered normal, are associated with an increased frequency of birth defects, toxaemia, Caesarean section and abnormal birth weights.[1] The best way to produce a stable blood sugar level, which does not swing too high or too low, is to eat frequent small meals that are high in soluble fibre and/or protein and are low in sugar.

WHAT TO EAT AND DRINK DURING PREGNANCY – AND WHAT TO AVOID

In the pages that follow, I will be giving you a lot of specific information about the foods and drinks that will help you create a healthy baby and keep your own immune system in top form. Before I get into details, though, it might not be a bad idea to look at a few basic principles that can guide you to sound nutrition during pregnancy:

- *Choose foods that are low in fat and sugar and/or high in fibre.* This is a good strategy at any time, but it is crucial during pregnancy. If you get many of your daily calories from sugar or the wrong kinds of fat, such as those in fried or greasy foods, then you're not getting the extra vitamins and minerals you must have to meet the needs of your developing foetus and to keep turning those EFAs into prostaglandins for your own immune system. You are also consuming anti-nutrients that block your body's metabolism of EFAs – so you're doing *double* damage to your immune system.

Fibre will protect you from that bane of pregnant women: constipation. It also helps to prevent swings in blood sugar levels.

- *Make sure you get enough calcium to fill both your own needs and the needs of your developing infant.* As your embryo develops into an infant, he needs plenty of calcium to build sound bones and teeth. At the same time, your own body needs about 800 mg of calcium a day (the equivalent of three glasses of milk) to maintain your own bones and teeth. So you will need to consume much more calcium than usual. If you don't add enough calcium to your diet, your baby will take what he needs from *your* teeth and bones.
- *Be wary of prepared, packaged and frozen foods, vitamin pills and mineral supplements, and all drugs: read labels carefully.* As we saw in Chapter 1, manufactured foods generally contain generous amounts of such anti-nutrients as partially hydrogenated vegetable oils, salt and sugar, so they really don't fit in with the principle of a low-fat, low-sugar diet. Manufactured foods also contain very little in the way of EFAs.

Vitamin pills and mineral supplements have to be approached with caution because, as we shall discover in a few pages, the wrong combinations can do more harm than good. And many drugs that are perfectly safe at other times have the potential to do damage to a developing foetus. Look for warnings on packages and in the literature that may come with your medication.

YOUR PREGNANCY DIET

Dairy products

If you are able to digest them, dairy products are the best source of calcium for both you and your unborn baby. They are generally terrific sources of protein as well, so when you eat dairy products, you are getting two essential nutrients for the price of one. Of course, whole-milk dairy products are high in fat, so low-fat versions are usually best.

I recommend four servings of dairy products, or the equivalent in high-calcium non-dairy foods, every day of your pregnancy. One serving of dairy products equals: 8 oz (225 g) of low-fat yoghurt, milk or cottage cheese; *or* 1½ oz (35 g) of low-sodium hard cheese.

You can substitute twice as much (3 oz/85 g) of soft white goat cheese (chèvre) for hard cheese, but because other kinds of soft cheese, such as brie, generally contain more water, you would have to eat twice as much to get the same amount of calcium. And this brings you up against the main problem of cheese: high fat content. Don't eat more than one serving of hard or goat cheese a day. It is a good idea to avoid full-fat cheeses altogether. As their name implies, they are virtually pure fat, and have very little nutritional value.

If you follow this plan, you will get 1100 mg of calcium each day from dairy products, plus a few hundred more from other foods. This is enough for your own and your baby's requirements, so you won't need to take a calcium supplement.

If you want to, you can double the calcium content of a single serving of yoghurt, milk or cottage cheese by mixing in 2½ fl. oz (70 ml) of non-fat dry milk powder. This adds 80 calories.

What if you have a lactose intolerance and can't digest dairy products? You can still get plenty of calcium from other foods. Here are five non-dairy equivalents to one serving of milk:

- 4 oz (115 g) canned fish with bones, such as sardines and pilchards (fresh fish won't give you the same amount of calcium unless you eat the bones).
- ½ oz (15 g) fresh kale or spring greens.
- 12 oz (340 g) dried beans – kidney beans, white or fava beans, or chickpeas.
- 3 oz (85 g) nuts. Almonds are highest in calcium. Walnuts and pecans are only fair. Peanuts don't count, since they aren't really nuts at all. Pistachios have little calcium.
- 3 oz seeds (85 g). Pumpkin seeds are excellent, sunflower fair to good.

Fish, poultry and meat

What you want to concentrate on here is lean and low-fat. You should eat at least 6 oz (170 g) of fish, poultry or lean meat, or a vegetarian equivalent, every day of your pregnancy.

Try to eat at least 12 oz/345 g (three 4 oz/115 g servings) of *fresh* oily, cold-water fish – salmon, tuna, mackerel, herring or sardines – every week. These fish are rich in omega-3 EFAs, which are vital for the developing nervous system of the foetus, and may also be important for its developing immune system.

Your own immune system will be working for two, so you need omega-3 EFAs to keep it running properly. Research has shown that, during pregnancy, a woman's immune system becomes slightly depressed, probably in order to keep her body from rejecting the developing embryo as if it were a parasite. It is all the more important, then, that you provide your immune system with as much nourishment as possible, so as not to weaken it any further!

Remember that fish vary in EFA content, and that processing and cooking can deplete or damage EFAs. White-fleshed fish such as sole or plaice contain few EFAs to start with. Fresh tuna, salmon and mackerel are excellent grilled or poached, or eaten cold in salads. Anchovies, herring and prawns are nice additions to salads, also. (I don't recommend the Japanese dishes sushi or sashimi, which are becoming increasingly popular. Both comprise raw fish, which can contain parasites – always cook fish before you eat it.) Mackerel can also be used in fish stews or soups. And one great luxury seafood – lobster – is a fair source of EFAs, so if you can, indulge yourself.

What about canned tuna? It's a fair source, especially the white albacore variety. But the oil used in the canning process is usually a vegetable oil low in omega-3s. Canning in water also lowers the EFA content, so canned fish is nutritionally inferior to fresh fish. If possible, grill, bake or poach your fish and grill or roast your poultry and meat. If you want to stir-fry or sauté, use a small amount of olive oil – one tablespoon (15 ml) will do for a family meal. I like olive oil better than vegetable oil for cooking because vegetable oils oxidize in heat to form harmful peroxides. Peroxides function like sparks to damage EFAs, not to mention your body cells, and may contribute to cancer. Olive oil resists peroxidation.

Olive oil also smokes easily, which means that you have to cook at a relatively low temperature. This helps preserve such nutrients as the B vitamins and vitamin C. Vitamin C, you will recall, is one of the essential vitamins that help your body turn EFAs into the prostaglandins that keep your immune system humming.

If you blanch some green leafy vegetable, such as spinach, in a frying pan first with a little water and some herbs, you can steam your fish or poultry – or even your meat – without fat in the same pan. This method also has the advantage of requiring a relatively low heat.

You needn't deprive yourself of red meat. It has received a bad press lately because even lean red meat contains more fat, especially more saturated fat, than fish or poultry. But red meat is rich in iron and zinc – both of which are important in helping your body metabolize EFAs – and are crucial nutrients for the developing foetus. Dark meat poultry, also under a cloud because it is fattier than white meat, is actually more nutritious than white meat. If you like it, go right ahead and eat it. During pregnancy, you need to be more concerned with supplying essential nutrients for both you and the developing foetus than with protecting yourself against future heart disease. The fat in meat can be included in the nutrients you need. The idea is to avoid *added* fat, which contains no other nutrients. So buy the leaner cuts of steak, such as rump steak, and trim the fat off; trim the skin off your dark meat chicken and turkey, if you wish, and enjoy the meat.

What if you are a vegetarian, or simply want some alternatives to fish, poultry or meat? There are many good non-meat sources of protein. You can substitute eggs, beans or nuts, using the following guidelines:

> *For 1 oz (30 g) meat:*
> 1 egg
> 1½ oz (40 g) cooked dried beans
> *For 3 oz (85 g) meat:*
> 2½ oz (65 g) nuts or seeds

Beans provide particularly good food value because they supply several essential nutrients and health factors besides protein, among them, as we have seen, calcium. Magnesium and copper in beans help your body process EFAs into the right prostaglandins. The fibre in beans helps prevent constipation. *You should eat at least 12 oz (340 g) of cooked beans a week.* If flatulence ('wind') is a problem, try soaking the beans overnight, discarding the soak water, and rinsing. This removes complex sugars that are the cause of flatulence for many. Or use bean curd (tofu), which is rendered more digestible by its processing. By pressing any type of bean through a strainer you can create a bean purée that is free of the skin. You lose fibre by doing this, but it will usually eliminate flatulence.

The protein value of beans is enhanced by combining them with whole grains. Any serious vegetarian must become familiar with Frances Moore Lappé's *Diet for a Small Planet* and its companion book, *Recipes for a Small Planet* by Ellen Buchman Ewald. Both focus on combining grains, seeds, nuts, beans and dairy products for high-protein meatless menus. A weakness of these books, though, is that they fail to pay equal attention to other nutrients.

Peanuts are not true nuts; they are pulses, like beans, and have a comparable protein value, although their fatty acid composition is inferior. Other seeds and nuts that are good sources of protein include sunflower, sesame and pumpkin seeds, and cashews and black walnuts.

Vegetables

These are an important source of vitamins C and A, both crucial for the foetus's development and for your own immune system. Vitamin C is essential for prostaglandin production, while vitamin A helps your immune system produce the lymphocytes that identify and kill enemy invaders. While you are pregnant, your own lymphocytes are thinking for two, so you want to keep them healthy. Your own skin, eyes and cells also need vitamin A. *You should eat four servings of vegetables every day of your pregnancy.*

The best vegetable sources for both vitamin C and vitamin A are tomatoes (considered a vegetable although it is officially a fruit of the vine), broccoli, asparagus, kale and peppers. Brussels sprouts and cauliflower are rich sources of vitamin C. Carrots, spinach and sweet potatoes are all excellent sources of vitamin A.

Vegetables are one of the most nutritious snack foods you can eat, and they contain almost no fat. Keep your refrigerator stocked with such vegetable crunchies as raw courgette and carrot sticks, cauliflower florets, pepper slices, cherry tomatoes and celery. Sweet, crisp, fresh mange-tout makes a delicious snack too, as do fresh young green beans.

Fruits

Oranges, grapefruit and strawberries are rich in vitamin C, a helper vitamin for EFAs. Apples and berries are good sources of fibre.

Bread, potatoes, pasta and cereals

These complex-cardohydrate foods are important sources of fibre and B vitamins. Vitamin B_6 helps turn EFAs into prostaglandins, to keep your immune system in tune. Complex carbohydrates also contain very little fat; this only appears in what is used to prepare them.

*Eat four servings a day from this group of foods.*One serving is equal to one of the following:

> 1 slice of bread
> 1½ oz (35 g) dry cereal
> ¾ oz (20 g) cooked cereal
> 1 medium potato

Choose whole-grain breads and cereals, and preferably those with no added sugar, such as whole-wheat shredded wheat or a homemade muesli (*see* recipe section in Chapter 10), as well as brown rice, barley, buckwheat groats (sometimes sold as kasha), whole-wheat pasta and our old friends, dried beans. (This makes beans a four-star food, offering you protein, calcium, and magnesium, as well as all the virtues of a complex carbohydrate.)

Read the ingredients list on any box of dry cereal, not only for sugar content but also for partially hydrogenated vegetable oil (an arch anti-nutrient) and salt.

Eat potatoes baked or boiled. Skip chips – they add unnecessary fat and they are a big source of anti-nutrient peroxides.

Spreads, toppings and condiments

Low-fat yoghurt, seasoned with chives and garlic, makes a delicious spread for potatoes. Yoghurt with dill or chives and/or garlic also goes well with most vegetables, whether cooked or raw. My tofu-based spread (see Chapter 10) is also delicious on potatoes and vegetables. Stay away from margarine and imitation butter, both full of the partially hydrogenated vegetable oil that is so destructive to your immune system. Butter, a source of vitamin A, is actually much less a dietary villain than these two highly touted substitutes.

Nut butters – almond, peanut, sesame – make great spreads for bread. Although they are high in calories, they are rich in minerals and EFAs. Be sure to get the unsalted variety.

If you want mayonnaise, use my recipe in Chapter 10, or buy a brand that's made with unhydrogenated soya oil. Don't use more than one tablespoon (15 ml) a day of the ordinary kind. My tofu mayonnaise is so nutritious that you can use as much as you want.

As we saw in Chapter 1, you can mix equal amounts of linseed oil and virgin olive oil as a base for salad dressing. Yoghurt or soft tofu mixed with vinegar and herbs work well, too. (See recipes in Chapter 10.) Many commercial salad dressings are poison to the immune system because they contain partially hydrogenated vegetable oil.

Seasonings and cooking oils

Avoid table salt altogether. According to the UK Recommended Dietary Allowances (UK RDA), the average person requires approximately 3500 mg of sodium a day, the equivalent of 9 g of table salt. (The US RDA for sodium is even lower – just 2000 mg, or 5 g of table salt.) However, as we have seen, many researchers believe that the average person ingests 10 to 20 times the amount of sodium necessary to maintain its balance in the body. The salt that is naturally contained in a balanced diet is all you need, even during pregnancy.

Among other things, salt helps to expand the volume of blood needed to nourish your placenta. But salt also contributes to fluid retention and may elevate your blood pressure – both common complications in the last months of pregnancy.

Cook without salt or soya sauce – there are excellent cookbooks that tell you how to prepare delicious meals without salt, using lemon juice, herbs and spices instead. Don't add salt at the table.

Whenever possible, ask restaurants to prepare your order without salt. Never add salt at the restaurant table, either. Avoid soya sauce and most other commercial sauces because of their high salt content.

Be very wary of packaged and prepared foods. Even those that appear to be healthy may contain large amounts of sodium. A single can or packet of soup may contain as much as 800 to 900 mg, almost one quarter of the daily salt dosage recommended by the UK RDA. Avoid tinned foods, or at least look for tinned vegetables and soups prepared without salt. *Always read labels carefully.*

WHAT YOU SHOULD AND SHOULD NOT DRINK

In addition to milk, which is a food as well as a drink, you will want to drink plenty of water during your pregnancy. *Do not drink chlorinated tap water. Drink only bottled spring water or well water that has been checked for purity.*

City tap water is always chlorinated and may contain a variety of environmental pollutants. In addition, it may contain lead leached in from the soldering on pipe joints. A study at the University of Perugia in Italy points to the possibility that substances produced by chlorination can damage genes.[2] Leached-in lead can damage the foetus's developing brain, leading to retardation and other problems. And environmental pollutants are potent anti-nutrients. Well water should be tested every few years, and if you have reason to doubt its purity, arrange with a water-testing service to examine it for microbes that may not be included in the usual tests.

Run water for three minutes to clear any that has been standing in the pipes before taking for food or drink. A charcoal filter on the tap is not effective against lead or chlorine, but can eliminate many chemical pollutants.

Bottled mineral waters are usually all right. Soda water should be made from filtered spring water and should contain no added salt.

Avoid any drink containing caffeine or alcohol. Any pregnant woman concerned about having a healthy baby should avoid such caffeine-containing drinks as coffee, tea, cocoa and chocolate milk, and fizzy drinks such as colas.

Pregnancy reduces the body's ability to metabolize caffeine by two-thirds. *When you are pregnant, one cup of coffee is as potent as three.* So if you drink two cups, the effect is the same as six.

Alcohol can lower a baby's birth weight and has been linked with neurological damage and delayed development in infants. It is also a powerful anti-nutrient that prevents your immune system from getting the prostaglandins it needs. Remember that a glass of wine, a bottle of beer and measure of spirits all contain approximately the same amount of pure alcohol – ½ fl. oz (14 ml). As for the new non-alcoholic beers, wines and ciders, most contain chemical additives whose effect is unknown.

The hard truth about soft drinks

Soft drinks such as colas, lemonade, squashes and the like can do nothing but harm to the developing foetus and to your own immune system. They contain sugar, an anti-nutrient, and no nutrients. Many low-calorie soft drinks contain NutraSweet, or aspartame, which has been proven, in laboratory studies, to harm the brains of young animals. If you drink it (or eat it in low-calorie desserts), you can't be sure it won't do the same to the foetus.

Moreover, studies suggest that one effect of aspartame may be to increase your own appetite for sugar-containing sweets – thus completely defeating their purpose and leading you to add more anti-nutrients to your diet.[3]

Many soft drinks also contain caffeine and phosphoric acid. Phosphoric acid blocks the absorption of calcium and magnesium by your intestines. This makes it an anti-nutrient that does harm to your immune system, because magnesium is the most important of the helper minerals that keeps prostaglandin production properly regulated. And prostaglandins, in turn, keep your immune system regulated.

ABOUT SMOKING

Don't smoke. Smoking doubles the risk of your baby having a low birth weight. According to the US National Academy of Sciences, underweight infants are more prone to serious diseases and more likely to have congenital conditions such as cerebral palsy, mental retardation, seizures and vision problems.

Harvard University researchers have discovered that, in babies whose mothers smoke, lung size is reduced by 10 per cent – a factor, according to the *New England Journal of Medicine*, that may contribute to the higher rate of respiratory disease in the children of smokers. Recent research has also found that maternal smoking in pregnancy may increase the risk of childhood cancer by 50 per cent.[4] If you are a smoker, don't resume smoking after your pregnancy ends. Numerous studies have documented the hazards of passive smoking (breathing someone else's cigarette smoke). For children, the immediate risk is an increase in the frequency, severity and duration of respiratory disease.[5]

CAN DRUGS BE TAKEN DURING PREGNANCY?

Not unless absolutely necessary, especially during the first three months. As we saw earlier, the first trimester is the most crucial period in terms of birth defects. But the developing foetus is at risk during your entire pregnancy. So avoid so-called 'recreational drugs' such as marijuana and cocaine, both of which have been linked to birth defects.

Stay away from such prescription and over-the-counter medical drugs as anti-histamines, aspirin, paracetamol, sleeping pills and painkillers. Avoid all anti-nausea medicines.

If you are prone to acne, beware of using Roaccutane (13-cis retinoic acid/isotretinoin), a prescription medication, both before your pregnancy and during the first three months. Women taking it have produced babies with marked abnormalities of the head and brain.

Read the label and the enclosed literature of every drug you think of taking while you are pregnant. Those considered dangerous should have a printed warning on the box and on an instruction sheet inside. But understand that drugs considered safe may not, in fact, *be* safe. Many warnings appear only after widespread side-effects have been discovered.

THE QUESTION OF NUTRITIONAL SUPPLEMENTS

You will need to take some supplements while you are pregnant. Studies have shown that the addition of certain vital nutrients in the right amount (often well above current government recommendations) can help reduce the risk of birth defects and protect a pregnancy from complications. But beware of taking megadoses of any supplement. In many cases, no one really knows what effect they will have on you or your unborn baby. What's more, when you take one vitamin or mineral, you could be interfering with your own – or your unborn baby's – ability to use some other vital nutrient. This is especially true with minerals. The commonly available antenatal multivitamin-and-mineral pills ignore this important fact. Their use may actually *worsen* deficiencies of key minerals such as zinc (crucial for EFA metabolism) and manganese.[6]

For both of these reasons, designing your own megadose programme – even if you have taken megadoses before your pregnancy without apparent harm – is like performing a potentially dangerous experiment on your unborn baby.

In the pages that follow, I will provide a proven, sensible programme of mineral and vitamin supplements that has been successfully followed by hundreds of my patients. I will also suggest specific supplements, and especially combinations of supplements, that you should avoid.

ESSENTIAL FATTY ACIDS

Most women don't get enough omega-3 EFAs. One result is an epidemic of dry skin and hair, a bonanza for the huge skin cream and hair-conditioner industries. Worse, though, as we saw in Chapter 1, EFA deficiency means an immune system that doesn't work as well as it should. Omega-3 EFAs are vitally important in regulating your own immune system and in helping your unborn baby's nervous system to develop properly. EFAs may also provide a special service in helping to prevent birth defects. And in animal studies, linseed oil, rich in both types of EFA (omega-6 and omega-3), has been shown to protect against cleft palate induced by a toxic drug.[7]

You *can* get enough EFAs – and the minerals and vitamins you need to help your body metabolize them and produce prostaglandins – from food alone, but it's not easy. What's more, there are no RDAs for EFAs yet, and you won't find them in most standard multivitamin formulas. In my experience, individual requirements for these crucial nutrients vary a lot, so you will want to keep yourself and your unborn baby well supplied.

I recommend a daily supplement of linseed oil or fish-oil extract. One or two tablespoons of food-grade linseed oil (available at healthfood shops and a few chemists) can be taken as a 'medicine', or used as salad oil. Don't use linseed oil for frying: heat plus air destroys its activity. If you prefer, you can take three 1-gram capsules of fish-oil extract (e.g. Max EPA) instead.

MINERALS

Calcium

As I explained on pages 20–21, calcium is an essential nutrient for both you and your unborn baby. Without it, your foetus will not be able to develop sound bones and teeth, and if you don't provide extra amounts for him, he will take what he needs from your bones. Food is the best source of calcium, as it is for most nutrients; but many women can't digest dairy products and may not wish to eat beans, canned fish, nuts and seeds, kale and/or spring greens every day. Enter the calcium supplement.

The tricky thing about calcium supplements is that they aren't always easily absorbed. Calcium carbonate, the cheapest form, comes from plain old chalk, oyster shells or dolomite. Calcium carbonate is very alkaline, so stomach acid is essential to make it soluble for absorption. It should always be taken with meals, because that's when the stomach secretes more acid to digest food. But even then, many women don't produce enough stomach acid to absorb this form of calcium very well.

This makes calcium citrate a good choice for a supplement. It consists of calcium from chalk that has been chemically compounded with citric acid, a chemical that occurs naturally in the body and helps supply energy. The result is so easily absorbed that any women can take it, even without food.

Normally, your body carefully regulates the amount of calcium you absorb, so that if you take more than you and your unborn baby need, you will excrete the extra calcium in your faeces. In a very few people, this regulation process doesn't work well, and those people are susceptible to kidney stones. But calcium citrate is so soluble that, when taken with plenty of magnesium, it will not precipitate kidney stone formation even if you are prone to them.

Therefore, if you are unable to eat the dairy or non-dairy food sources of calcium outlined on pages 20–21 under 'Dairy products', you should take 750–1000 mg of a calcium citrate supplement each day. A good time to take calcium is at bedtime, so that you avoid blocking absorption of other key minerals (*see* list, p. 37). Also, blood calcium levels tend to fall overnight, so you help your bones more by taking calcium just before sleep.

In some people, calcium may cause constipation. This can be easily corrected by adding 100–200 mg of magnesium a day to the amounts recommended in the next section. The possibility of this minor annoyance is no reason to deprive your unborn baby of one of the most important nutrients you can give him.

Magnesium

This mineral is important both in its own right and as a balance to calcium intake. It is stored in your bones, where it helps them retain their calcium. If your magnesium supplies are low, you will lose more of the calcium you take in, making less available for you and your unborn baby. *For maximum effectiveness, most authorities recommend that you balance calcium and magnesium in a two-to-one ratio.* This means that you should take one part of magnesium for every two parts of calcium. If you take 1000 mg of calcium each day, or get that much in food, you should be getting 500 mg of magnesium. Some women, though, need twice as much magnesium or more – an amount equal to or greater than the amount of calcium they take in each day. If you are irritable, constipated, or easily fatigued, have trouble sleeping or get muscle cramps easily, you may have a magnesium deficiency.

Perhaps even more important, magnesium is an important nutrient in your unborn baby's development. A recent West German study of 1000 pregnant women found that those who took magnesium supplements of 400 mg a day produced babies with higher birth weights and slightly higher Apgar scores. (This is a 10-point index of vitality and alertness given to babies immediately and five minutes after birth.) Overall, these women also had fewer spontaneous abortions (i.e. miscarriages) and suffered less from such complications of pregnancy as toxaemia.[8]

Yet the US RDA for magnesium is only 300 mg, raised to only about 450 mg for pregnant women. Many supplements, particularly multivitamins and mineral supplements, simply don't contain enough magnesium for a pregnant woman.

It's hard to get enough magnesium in a typical diet, which is short on such magnesium-rich foods as beans and nuts. In addition, stress depletes the supplies of magnesium your bones and cells do contain. I frequently encounter magnesium deficiency, even in women who believe they are well nourished.

I recommend a magnesium supplement to all pregnant patients. In addition to the amount you may be getting in food to balance your calcium intake, you will want to take from 300 to 400 mg each day to counter any possible deficiency. The amount depends on your weight:

100 lb (7 stone 2)	300 mg
120 lb (8 stone 8)	360 mg
140 lb (10 stone)	420 mg
160 lb (11 stone 6)	400 mg

If cramps, irritability or insomnia persist, you should double the dosage. For a woman with normal kidney function, and for her unborn baby, the danger of overdosing on magnesium is practically non-existent. At worst, too much may cause diarrhoea, at which point you can reduce the supplement.

Should you take a supplement that combines calcium and magnesium? While such preparations are increasingly popular, most of them rely on calcium carbonate and magnesium oxide, a combination that may be difficult for your body to absorb. Magnesium oxide, like calcium carbonate, dissolves only in stomach acid – and, as we saw above, many women don't produce enough stomach acid to do the job. But there is another hitch, as well – the calcium carbonate may block absorption of the magnesium oxide. In any case, calcium–magnesium tablets are often so tightly compacted that they pass intact right through your digestive system.

I recommend taking calcium and magnesium separately: calcium in the form of calcium citrate, and magnesium as magnesium citrate or magnesium chloride.

There are a number of other minerals you should take as supplements in order to ensure that you are getting adequate amounts.

Iron

This is needed by your unborn baby in the development of his brain and to build his blood cells, including the crucial white blood cells of the immune system. If you don't supply extra iron, he'll take what he needs from supplies that your own body needs. And it's very hard to get enough of this essential mineral to meet the needs of pregnancy from your food alone. That's why most antenatal vitamin supplements contain 20 mg of iron a day, often in combination with folic acid (*see below*).

Zinc

This element is absolutely crucial in the development of your baby's thymus, the most important organ in the immune system. The thymus is a gland in which the T-cells, the brain of the immune system, will be produced and trained to do their job properly. Zinc also stimulates growth. And, like iron and calcium, if you don't supply extra amounts, the growing foetus will take what it needs from your own body's essential stores.

As we shall see, your body's ability to use zinc is affected by other vitamins and minerals. A recent British study showed that the usual antenatal multivitamin supplements actually cause a 30 per cent *reduction* in the amount of zinc a pregnant woman is able to absorb.[9]

Copper

Another mineral that is needed by the foetus for the proper development of its immune system and brain. Yet even non-pregnant women usually get much less copper than the US RDA, which is 1.6 mg. A study done at Virginia Polytechnic Institute in the United States found that pregnant women eating food of their own choice are actually in negative copper balance (they use more copper than they consume); their zinc and copper status was improved significantly by supplementation.[10] In addition, *high-EFA foods – beans, nuts, seafood, liver and kidney – are also good sources of iron, zinc and copper.*

Manganese

Needed to help prevent birth defects,[11] it is found in whole grains and nuts, but the iron supplements you take during pregnancy will block its absorption.

Trace elements

These are minerals that your body needs in amounts less than 1 milligram a day. *Selenium* helps prevent birth defects, cancer and heart disease. *Chromium* helps your body's insulin to keep your blood sugar stabilized, an important job during pregnancy because hyperglycaemia and hypoglycaemia can harm your baby (*see* p. 19). You donate a lot of chromium to your baby during pregnancy, and with each succeeding pregnancy, your chromium depletion increases. *Iodine* is essential for the development of your unborn baby's thyroid gland. Iodine deficiency during pregnancy produces a mentally retarded baby. Luckily, seafood is a rich source of iodine. *If you don't eat three servings of seafood a week, you need an iodine supplement.*

VITAMINS

A strong argument for taking vitamin supplements during pregnancy is provided by studies that link vitamin deficiencies to birth defects. And you *can* have a vitamin deficiency even if you are getting the RDA, which may not be large enough to protect you and your developing baby during your pregnancy. This is particularly true of the B vitamins. Several studies have shown that multivitamin supplements taken throughout pregnancy could be an important step in preventing such birth defects as *spina bifida*, in which the spinal vertebrae are incompletely formed; other spinal defects; and cleft palate.[12]

One B vitamin, *Vitamin B6* (also known as *pyridoxine*), is important in helping EFAs make the prostaglandins that regulate your immune system. It is marginally deficient in 50 per cent of pregnant women.[13] The current US RDA for vitamin B6 for pregnant women is 2.6 mg a day, yet a recent study at the University of Florida showed that a dose of 20 mg or more, about *ten times* the US RDA, may be needed just to maintain normal blood levels during pregnancy. And according to the same study, 10 to 20 mg of vitamin B6 a day produced newborns with 10 per cent higher Apgar scores than those attained by babies whose mothers took less than 10 mg a day.[14]

An added benefit of vitamin B6 is that it may help prevent hand pain, a surprisingly common problem in pregnancy. The *Journal of the Canadian Medical Association* reports that up to 25 per cent of pregnant women suffer from *carpal tunnel syndrome*: pain and tingling in the palms and fingers and weakness in the thumbs. Several other studies, including one at the University of Washington, have linked this syndrome with vitamin B6 deficiency. Women with carpal tunnel syndrome may need 100 to 500 mg a day to correct their deficiency.[15]

Isn't it true that vitamin B6 is toxic in high doses? True – a report in the *New England Journal of Medicine* told of a few people who developed reversible nerve damage after consuming exceptionally high doses of vitamin B6 – 2000 mg or more a day – for several months. At this megadose level, it appears that vitamin B6 can actually block its own effect in the body. The doses I usually recommend to pregnant women – 25 mg a day (about ten times the US RDA) – are, however absolutely non-toxic. On the contrary, most women need this amount to help counteract environmental pollutants such as herbicides, which interfere with the body's ability to use vitamin B6.

Folic acid, part of the B-complex of vitamins, helps your body produce white blood cells, without which your immune system has no army with which to fight germs. What's more, folic-acid deficiency causes anaemia. Your body's folic acid requirements double during pregnancy, and in my experience folic acid deficiencies are very common in pregnant women who don't take supplements. It has also been found that folic-acid supplementation may prevent babies from developing spina bifida.

Vitamins A and C are essential co-factor vitamins in the metabolism of EFAs, so you need good supplies to keep your immune system well regulated.

High doses of vitamin C don't appear to do any harm to developing babies (contrary to one report, they will not produce babies so conditioned to high levels of vitamin C that they get scurvy without them). But too much vitamin A can cause birth defects. If you're even *thinking* about getting pregnant, don't take over 10,000 IU (international units) of vitamin A a day.

Vitamin E in doses of 200 IU per day (about five times the US RDA) appears to be useful in preventing spontaneous abortion (miscarriage).[16] *Choline*, sometimes classified as a B vitamin, should not be taken in pregnancy, nor should lecithin supplements, which are a common source of choline. Studies with pregnant rats show that maternal use of lecithin affects the developing brain cells of the foetus, producing abnormal behaviour in the offspring.[17] The reason is probably related to the body's use of choline in making a *neurotransmitter* (nerve chemical) called acetylcholine. Higher than normal levels of such neurotransmitters in the foetal brain may cause permanent neurological changes. It is likely that other natural substances used by the body to make other neurotransmitters may also be toxic to the developing brain. These would consist primarily of individual amino acids, such as tryptophan, tyrosine, phenylalanine and glutamic acid, which are used to control appetite, mood, pain and insomnia. The toxic effect of aspartame (NutraSweet) on very young animals probably shares a similar mechanism, because NutraSweet consists of the amino acids phenylalanine and glutamic acid.

TAKING VITAMINS AND MINERALS

Can you take minerals and vitamins in multimineral and multivitamin supplements, or even in a single multivitamin-and-mineral tablet or capsule? This is the form in which many people are accustomed to getting their minerals and vitamins. They are widely sold and are appealing because they seem to simplify the whole process of taking supplements. But, as with calcium and magnesium, there are many combinations of minerals, and of vitamins and minerals, that should not be taken at the same time. Calcium can block the body's ability to absorb zinc, iron and copper. Zinc interferes with the absorption of iron, and vice versa. High doses of vitamin C and/or zinc will block absorption of selenium. And too much zinc can deplete the body's copper and manganese levels. The combination of copper and vitamins B_1 (thiamin), B_{12} and C may produce a substance known as a 'vitamin B_{12}

analogue' – a chemical similar to B_{12} but which, in fact, blocks the action of B_{12} in the body.[18] Both you and the developing foetus need B_{12} to make blood cells – including those all-important immune-system white blood cells – and to help your brain and nerves work properly.

And because the RDAs of most vitamins don't account for your body's special needs during pregnancy, many of the most popular multivitamin and mineral supplements, including the most-prescribed antenatal supplements, simply do not provide high enough doses to be effective.

What's more, some supplements contain undesirable elements. Bioflavonoids are popular these days, and are included in some vitamin C supplements. Unfortunately, the bioflavonoid *rutin* can be converted in the intestine into another bioflavonoid, *quercetin*, that can damage chromosomes – leading to potential genetic damage in a developing foetus.[19] You'd be smart to avoid bioflavonoids during pregnancy, especially during the critical first three months.

During pregnancy, I recommend taking each vitamin and mineral separately, and in combinations that will not interfere with absorption or use by the body. The following provides a simple, safe, effective programme of daily dosages, with a schedule that will allow maximum effectiveness for each supplement. (You will take most supplements with meals to give your body the best chance to absorb them.)

ESSENTIAL FATTY ACIDS

As a liquid: 1 to 2 tablespoons (15–30 ml) of food-grade linseed oil per day. To maximize absorption, take right before or after a meal. Or use in dressings on salads, vegetables and pasta. *Do not fry with it; high heat and air destroy EFAs.* You may substitute 1 teaspoon to 1 tablespoon (5–15 ml) of cod-liver oil.

In capsules: Three to six 1-gram capsules of fish-oil extract per day. (It will require 15 to 30 linseed oil capsules a day to equal 1 to 2 tablespoons of linseed oil.) MaxEPA is a standard brand.

VITAMINS

Vitamin   *Daily dosage*

A   10,000 units, or 1 tablespoon cod-liver oil, or one 8-ounce glass carrot juice (best choice)

B complex

B_1	10 mg
B_2 (riboflavin)	10 mg
B_3 (nicotinic acid)	100 mg
B_6 (pyridoxine)	10–30 mg
B_{12}	10–20 micrograms (μg)
Folic acid	800 μg
Pantothenic acid	200 mg
Biotin	300 μg

C   1000 mg

D   400 international units (IU), or 1 teaspoon (5 ml) cod-liver oil

E   400 IU, as d-alpha-tocopherol (its most active form)

MINERALS

Mineral	Daily Dosage
Calcium	750–1000 mg (calcium citrate)
Magnesium	300–600 mg (magnesium citrate or magnesium chloride)
Iron	30–60 mg, with food and vitamin C
Zinc	15–20 mg The best form is zinc citrate or zinc picolinate. Do *not* take with iron.
Manganese	5 mg Do *not* take with iron.
Copper	2 mg, with vitamin C.
Selenium	200 μg The best form is selenomethionine. Do *not* take with zinc or vitamin C.
Chromium	400 μg Take the GTF (glucose-tolerance factor) form because, bound to an organic complex, the chromium is easily absorbed.
Iodine	200 μg *only* if you *do not* eat seafood

WHEN TO TAKE WHAT

The following list will enable you to get the most value from your supplements.

BREAKFAST   *Vitamins:* A, B_1, B_2 (riboflavin), B_3 (nicotinic acid), B_6 (pyridoxine), folic acid, pantothenic acid, biotin, C, D
Minerals: iron, copper

LUNCH   *Vitamin:* E
Minerals: magnesium, selenium, chromium, iodine

DINNER   *Vitamin:* B_{12}
Minerals: zinc, manganese

BEDTIME   *Mineral:* calcium citrate

HOW FOOD AND SUPPLEMENTS CAN OVERCOME MORNING SICKNESS

Eat for nausea? That sounds like a contradiction, and no one is exactly sure why it works, but it often does. Time and time again, I have found that my patients have been able to stop morning sickness by doing exactly what they had been avoiding – eating, and eating well.

Eat small meals of low-fat foods. Fats will make your nausea worse. Wholewheat bread or oatmeal, salt-free crackers, rice, fish and vegetables are good choices. Meat, nuts, fruit and dairy products may contribute to your nausea.

If food alone doesn't clear up the nausea, and the problem is severe enough to limit weight gain, I turn to supplements, which nearly always work. My own theory is that poor nutrition and hormonal changes produce deficiencies of vitamin B_6 (pyridoxine) and vitamin K, which interfere with the activity of key enzymes that regulate the function of the nausea centre in the brain. Patients I have been treating nutritionally before their pregnancies uniformly report less nausea than in earlier pregnancies. If I don't see a patient until she's already pregnant, urgent measures may be needed.

When Linda came to me during her pregnancy because she was nauseated and vomiting frequently, I gave her an initial dose of 100 mg of vitamin B_6, followed by an injection of 10 mg of vitamin K. She went home and, under my orders, continued taking 100 mg of B_6 a day for a week. By the end of the week, Linda's nausea had cleared up. The rest of her pregnancy was normal.

For morning sickness, I recommend 100 to 200 mg of B_6 and 10 mg of vitamin K a day. Occasionally, more than 200 mg of vitamin B_6 a day is necessary, but this amount should only be taken under a doctor's supervision. I also give patients an initial injection of vitamin K, which works in a day or two. Taken by mouth, the vitamin K takes somewhat longer to produce results – about ten days.

EXERCISE DURING PREGNANCY

It is fashionable today for young mothers-to-be to start or continue with a programme of strenuous aerobic exercise during pregnancy. *Exercise is beneficial, but I think there is a danger in strenuous exercise during pregnancy.*

In animal studies, internal temperatures in the range of 102° F (38.9 C) increase the frequency of birth defects. Strenuous aerobic exercise, especially distance running, can easily raise body temperature to that level, imperilling your health and that of your unborn child. If you are already an experienced runner, plan to keep your distances under six miles a day during pregnancy. If you have not been active before, your best bets for exercise are swimming, stationary cycling or brisk walking. Start with short times or distances, and always warm up before you start. (A brisk walk is good, as are leg-lifts and 'bicycling' with your legs in the air while lying on your back. These last two exercises strengthen your abdominal muscles and your legs as well as warming you up.)

If you feel comfortable, you can exercise right through pregnancy. But remember – don't try to set any records. Exercise only as long as it feels comfortable. Anyone with a medical history of miscarriages should consult a doctor before beginning any exercise programme.

LEARNING TO RELAX

When you're pregnant, your body is working full time to create another human being. Adding to this the challenges and demands of a home, a career and the nurture of other children, if you have them, can be very taxing to mind and body.

Stress, whether physical or emotional, can do harm during pregnancy. The increased adrenalin secreted during psychological stress can decrease the flow of blood to the foetus, particularly if stress is prolonged. In experiments, stressed animals have delivered litters of lower-than-average birth weight.

Make a conscious effort to take time out for yourself and to counter stress with calming meditation and relaxation exercises. Here are some brief but effective breathing and relaxation exercises that my patients use.

BREATHING EXERCISE

1 Stand with your arms at your sides.
2 Breathe out as much as you can through your nose.
3 To force more air out, contract your abdominal muscles strongly.
4 Breathe in slowly through both nostrils.
5 Fill the lower part of your lungs by letting your abdominal muscles relax so your abdomen bulges out.
6 Keep breathing in and fill the middle part of your lungs by expanding your rib cage.
7 Finish breathing in as you fill the upper part of your lungs by raising your shoulders.
8 Breathe out slowly.
9 Let your rib cage contract.
10 Finally, tighten your diaphragm and abdominal muscles to empty your lungs of air.
Repeat three times.

RELAXATION EXERCISE

The purpose of this exercise is to stretch muscles that most people keep chronically tense. This promotes relaxation.
1 Carry out the breathing exercise above.
2 Sit comfortably in a chair that supports your arms. Notice how much tension is present in your shoulders. Pull your shoulders down towards your hips, feeling their movement. Let them return to a neutral position and feel how much more relaxed they are. Let this feeling of relaxation travel from your shoulders down both arms into your hands.
3 Open your hands as wide as you can. Stretch your fingers. Feel each finger pulling away from every other finger and from the centre of your palm. Do this for 5 seconds, and then stop, relax and let your hands assume a natural position. Feel how relaxed they are.
4 Now pay attention to your legs, from your feet up to your hips. Feel how much tension is in them. Stretch your legs out, raising your heels 3 or 4 inches (7.5–10 cm) from the floor. Begin the stretch in your heels and pull through your knees to your hips. Point your toes gently towards your face. Feel the stretch in your legs and then let them relax. Feel how relaxed they are. Let the relaxation spread up your thighs and into your lower back.
5 Pay attention to your jaws. Feel how tense they are. Keeping your mouth closed, push your chin down towards your chest. Let your tongue hang naturally in the middle of your mouth; don't push it down, or up to the roof of

your mouth. Feel the muscles in your cheeks stretching. Now relax your jaws. Feel how relaxed they are.

6 Turn your attention to your forehead and eyes. Close your eyes gently, just letting your lids drop. Imagine a hand caressing your forehead, starting at your eyebrows and caressing upward, smoothing all the wrinkles and continuing over the top of your head, down the back of your neck, and into your shoulders.

7 Now repeat Steps 2 to 6.

Note: Natural childbirth classes often include relaxation exercises, and these can be used when you feel tense. However, the breathing exercises you learn in natural childbirth classes are intended for use during labour; they won't help calm you during pregnancy.

THE LAST WORD: SLEEP

Pregnant women need the health-promoting rest of a good night's sleep. But sleeping pills may cause birth defects, and the amino acid *tryptophan*, otherwise a safe, non-chemical sleep aid, can be carcinogenic (i.e. cancer-causing) in a pregnant woman's body. Why? Because your body maintains a high level of the female hormone *oestrogen* during pregnancy, and oestrogen acts to convert tryptophan into a carcinogen.

Take calcium citrate and/or magnesium citrate or chloride. Calcium and magnesium encourage sleep. If your bedtime calcium supplement doesn't help you sleep, try taking magnesium at bedtime. If you don't use a calcium supplement because you get all the calcium you need from food, take just the magnesium at bedtime. Keep raising the magnesium dose until you get diarrhoea or a good night's sleep.

From Birth to Six Months – Breastfeeding to Create High Health

3

Should a busy working mother take the time and trouble to breastfeed her infant? Despite the convenience of bottles and formulas, modern research has shown that the answer is a resounding *yes!* Studies show that bottle-fed infants get sick more often than those who are breastfed, because the immune systems of newborn infants are not yet able to perform at peak levels. Breast milk contains substances that will protect them against allergies and many of the infections common to bottle-fed babies. Other substances help their immune systems to develop. What's more, recent evidence suggests that breastfeeding may produce straighter teeth than bottle-feeding. And, as a dividend, breastfeeding offers some decided benefits to the new mother. It helps her recover more quickly from childbirth, it may protect her from breast cancer later in life, and it offers her some protection against conceiving again.

For the first six months of an infant's life, breast milk is the optimum food. For that reason, *I recommend that a new mother breastfeed as much as possible during her baby's first six months of life. Fulltime breastfeeding is best, but part-time breastfeeding is the next-best thing you can do.* There are a few exceptions, which I shall discuss later (p. 50).

Breastfeeding while holding down a fulltime job is difficult – it demands planning, flexibility and the sympathetic cooperation of a care giver. To breastfeed fulltime, you will also need the right conditions at work. But the benefits for your new baby are so substantial that I urge you to consider attempting it anyway.

For a variety of reasons, some women are unable to breastfeed at all. If you have this problem, you can still protect your baby to some extent. Although no formula available today can provide the same protection as breast milk, it is possible to make up for some of the deficiencies of formulas with supplements, especially after the first three months.

In the pages that follow, I will show you what breastfeeding can do for your baby and for you. I will also outline complete feeding programmes to provide the best possible nutrition for your newborn baby, whether you are able to breastfeed fulltime, parttime or not at all.

WHAT BREAST MILK CAN DO FOR YOUR BABY

A DIRECT BOOST TO THE IMMUNE SYSTEM

Infants' immune systems are immature. They start functioning as soon as the babies are born, but their lymphocytes are naïve – they have not yet met any of the thousands of different germs, bacteria, fungi and other invaders they will encounter in the children's lifetime. They can respond to foreign bodies, but because they must start from scratch for each one, they are slow.

A newborn infant's lymphocytes are also not yet capable of making all the different kinds of antibodies she needs. They acquire that ability slowly over her first year of life. The last one they begin to make is the *IgA antibody*, which performs a crucial service: coating her intestinal and respiratory tracts, thus protecting them against infection. Because their bodies can't yet make the IgA antibody, infants under a year are particularly prone to intestinal-tract infections.

Fortunately, a newborn infant still has her mother's antibodies in her blood. They will augment her defences during her first three months. After that, they are gone, but by that time her immune system has had a taste of the outside world and can handle some defensive jobs on its own. But because she still can't make that key IgA molecule, her intestinal tract remains vulnerable. Some of the special substances in breast milk are uniquely designed to protect your infant's intestinal tract from infection until she is ready to do it herself. Others enhance her overall defences, while still others help her immune system strengthen and mature.

Let's take a look at these substances.

● *Bifidus growth factor.* Bifidus is a lactobacillus, a good bacteria that guards against intestinal infection. It turns lactose, or milk sugar, into lactic acid, and lactic acid in turn discourages the growth of yeast, harmful bacteria and parasites in the intestinal tract. Because of a growth factor in breast milk, bifidus thrives in the intestines of breastfed babies. But because cow's milk contains no such factor, bifidus does not grow in the intestines of bottle-fed babies.

As an older infant's IgA levels rise, she doesn't need as much bifidus. When she starts to eat solid food, bifidus gradually disappears from her intestinal tract.

● *Immunoglobins.* These are antibodies that protect your infant against a wide range of infections, particularly in her intestinal tract. They help make up for her inability to produce IgA antibodies.

● *Interferon.* Genetically engineered interferon is being used experimentally against cancer and other diseases. Your body makes small amounts of it naturally, and it is contained in breast milk. It combats viruses that can cause intestinal infections, preventing them from replicating and spreading the infection.

● *Enzymes.* Human milk (and only human milk) contains an enzyme that breaks down the fat in the milk to form individual, free fatty acids. These free fatty acids (both essential and non-essential) inhibit the growth of parasites in the intestine. They are especially effective at killing off *Giardia lamblia*, a one-celled parasite that is a common – and often unrecognized – cause of diarrhoea in infants. Breastfed infants are more resistant to *Giardia* infection than those who are bottle-fed. Heating, by the way, rapidly destroys this important enzyme.

● *Iron and lactoferrin* Most infant formulas contain iron, up to two to three times more than breast milk. But the iron in formulas is not easily absorbed by a very young infant, and intestinal bacteria thrive on the unabsorbed iron in her digestive tract. This is where lactoferrin comes in. It is a protein in breast milk that combines with iron to make it more easily absorbed by an infant. What's more, lactoferrin inhibits the growth of bacteria to give your baby double protection.

Between three and six months of age, an infant becomes more able to absorb iron. From six to ten months, she may need extra iron if she is exclusively breastfed, because breast milk may not contain enough. By this time, as her maturing immune system begings to produce IgA antibodies, she will be able to defend herself against bacterial infections in her intestines.

● *Zinc.* Infant formulas are also usually fortified with zinc, but, as with iron, the zinc in breast milk is more easily absorbed by an infant. Zinc is essential for the development of the thymus gland, in which T-cells are 'educated' for their key role as the 'mind' of the immune system: recognizing invaders and calling out the troops to do battle.

● *Anti-oxidants.* In Chapter 1, we described the crucial role of the 'anti-oxidant defence system' in protecting white blood cells when they burn germs. At such times, the white blood cells become tiny furnaces. They need anti-oxidant protection in order not to burn themselves up. And germ-burning white blood cells also give off free radicals, the 'sparks' that can damage cell membranes, chromosomes and enzymes. Anti-oxidants quench those sparks.

● *Selenium and taurine.* These are two key anti-oxidants that are contained in breast milk but are not added in sufficient amount to formulas. Breast milk contains three times more *selenium* than formulas. Studies have shown that, when infants are breastfed for two to three months and then switched to formula, the levels of selenium in their blood go down.[1] But infants who are breastfed even part-time for up to a year keep high levels of selenium in their blood. The selenium content of human milk, moreover, is influenced by the mother's own selenium levels.[2]

By the time they are a year old, bottle-fed infants begin to get selenium in their solid food. But from three to nine months, they suffer a temporary deficiency that can have dramatic consequences. Selenium-deficient animals are susceptible to infection because their white blood cells simply don't survive as well without anti-oxidant protection. Among humans, breastfed infants hardly ever get chronic diarrhoea, whereas bottle-fed infants frequently do. The ratio is 100 to 1: for every breastfed baby who gets chronic diarrhoea, 100 bottle-fed babies get it.

In addition to its role as an anti-oxidant, *taurine* plays a critical role in brain development and digestion. Your body manufactures it from dietary protein, but your infant's body isn't able to do that yet. Taurine is not found in cow, soya or goat's milk, and has only recently begun to be added to formulas

Anti-oxidants such as selenium and taurine are probably also important in preventing respiratory-tract infections, but these have not yet been studied as thoroughly as digestive-tract infections. The combined surface area of both systems – one of which filters all the air your child breathes, while the other filters all her food – is enormous. An adult's intestinal tract alone contains a surface equal to that of a tennis court. White blood cells protect this huge surface area against the infections to which it is continuously exposed – and anti-oxidants protect the white blood cells.

● *GLA.* In Chapter 1, we found out how the body converts EFAs into prostaglandins, chemicals that in turn regulate the activity of the cells in the immune system. Prostaglandins are especially important to the health of lymphocytes. Enzymes in your liver convert the key omega-6 EFA, linoleic acid (LA), into GLA, an important intermediate step on the road to prostaglandin production. But the immature livers of newborns and infants don't produce enough of the key enzyme to be able to make this conversion. As a result, bottle-fed infants are more prone to allergies. Breastfeeding bypasses the whole problem by supplying GLA directly to your infant.

ANTI-ALLERGY PROTECTION

Because breast milk contains GLA and other EFAs, breastfeeding can actually delay the onset of food allergies as well as other allergic symptoms such as rashes and nasal discharges.[3]

On the other hand, cow's milk in the first year and the too-early feeding of solid food can both precipitate allergies. Why? Because an infant's intestinal tract is porous; it can't screen out the big molecules that cause allergies. This is why infants under a year old are particularly susceptible to food allergies, and why you should not feed an infant wheat, cow's milk, fish or egg whites during her first year of life. It takes 6–12 months for an infant's intestinal tract to develop the ability to screen out allergenic molecules.

Jonathan's mother brought him to me when he was two. His family was very allergy-prone: both his parents suffered from hay fever and asthma, and his older brothers each had multiple allergies and one had eczema. Jonathan's mother had breastfed him for a whole year, and during that time, he had not had a single allergy. But when he began to eat solid food, he, too, developed allergic symptoms, in the form of nasal congestion and eczema. Even so, his symptoms were much milder than those of his brothers, who had been bottle-fed.

Jonathan might have avoided allergies altogether if his mother had been better nourished. She was very prone to colds, and her hair was dull and limp. All this, with the number and severity of her own allergic symptoms, suggested an EFA deficiency that had undoubtedly affected the quality of her breast milk, making it less protective for Jonathan than it might otherwise have been.

To give Jonathan's mother EFA protection, I started her on 1 tablespoon (15 ml) of linseed oil and 1 teaspoon (5 ml) of cod-liver oil daily. After six weeks, her hair became glossy and lustrous; that winter she went without a cold and, as I expected, had fewer allergic symptoms.

For Jonathan, I prescribed 200 mg of vitamin C, 1 teaspoon (15 ml) of linseed oil and 1 teaspoon (15 ml) of cod-liver oil, all given at once in his orange juice each day. After four weeks, he was no longer congested and sniffling, and his skin had become smooth to the touch. His hair looked shinier and he himself was happier and more alive.

A breastfeeding mother, then, needs to keep herself well nourished, particularly in terms of EFAs. If you have a family history of allergies, I would suggest that you *breastfeed until your child weans herself.* Delay the introduction of infant formula as long as you can; try for six months of fulltime breastfeeding.

Ongoing research at Harvard Medical School and Boston Children's Hospital in Massachusetts suggests that giving formula at too early an age to allergy-prone infants who are also being breastfed can increase the risk of intestinal inflammation. The immune-stimulating effect of mother's milk makes the *very young* infant more likely to mount a strong immune response to any foreign protein that enters her intestine, whether the protein comes from an invading bacteria or from food. Dr W. Allan Walker, an immunologist who heads the Combined Program in Pediatric Gastroenterology and Nutrition at Harvard, advises mothers not to mix breast and formula feeding if there is a history of milk allergy in their parents or siblings. If a mixed feeding programme is necessary, Walker suggests the use of a hydrolyzed infant formula that is partially predigested and less allergenic.

Whether Walker's warnings apply to the first few weeks of life or the first few months is not known, and the final outcome of his research is still pending. As it now stands, this research is another piece of evidence against the use of formula feedings in the first few months of life.

Other important pieces of advice are: *Be sure that you are getting plenty of EFAs, especially the omega-3s*; and *start giving your baby linseed, walnut or cod-liver oil at six months. (See* p. 54 for tips on giving linseed oil to babies.) This last is good advice for any mother, whether or not her child is susceptible to allergies.

WHAT BREASTFEEDING CAN DO FOR YOU

Breastfeeding is a terrific way to tighten the bond between you and your newborn because it calls for the kind of holding and touching that helps sensitize you to each other. As you watch your baby breastfeed, you are going to make eye contact with her – an important part of the growing closeness between the two of you. All this can be done fairly well with a bottle, although women who breastfeed often report intense internal sensations that can make them even more responsive to their infants.

A bottle can't help your body recover more quickly from childbirth. Nursing triggers the secretion of *oxytocin*, a hormone that makes the uterus contract, helping it return to its normal state more quickly than it would otherwise.

Breastfeeding may also protect you against developing breast cancer later in life. Scientists at the Fred Hutchinson Cancer Research Center in Seattle, Washington, report that, in a study they carried out, women who breastfed had half the risk of developing breast cancer compared with those who didn't.

As long as you breastfeed, you will be somewhat less fertile than usual – although, unfortunately, you can't really rely on this factor as a contraceptive. Breastfeeding elevates your body's levels of *prolactin*, a hormone that tends to inhibit ovulation – but not 100 per cent! (One contraceptive method *not* to use is an IUD ('coil'). We now know that women who have an IUD inserted while breastfeeding run ten times the risk of perforation of the uterus than those who have one inserted after their infants are weaned.)

As a final bonus, fulltime breastfeeding burns about 250 calories a day, the equivalent of a three-mile run. This can help offset the fact that you will still be eating more than you normally would. You can cut the amount of food you ate while you were pregnant by 25 per cent (from 2500 calories a day to about 1900). As a result, while you are breastfeeding you should begin to lose about half a pound a week.

Although you may be eager to lose more than 2 lb a month, I don't recommend it. A strict diet may jeopardize the quality of your breast milk, with potential repercussions for your baby's health. In a University of Utah study, researchers observed 12 women who breastfed for ten weeks after giving birth. On a 1500-calorie-a-day diet, all the women complained of fatigue and said their babies didn't seem satisfied with their feedings. In addition, all the mothers produced fewer than the 22–24 fluid ounces of milk a day that most well-fed mothers produce.

Fat-soluble pollutants are another reason to steer clear of diets. Because of pervasive pollution of the environment, nearly all of us have measurable levels of such poisons as DDT, chlordane, dieldrin and even PCBs in our blood. The toxins accumulate in fatty tissue, including breast tissue. But as long as you don't fast or lose weight rapidly, they will stay in your own fatty tissue and won't accumulate in your breast milk. Sudden weight loss – a melting away of fat – will release these poisons into your blood, and into your milk.

WHAT SUPPLEMENTS SHOULD YOU TAKE WHILE BREASTFEEDING?

As nutritional insurance, you should continue with the supplements recommended for pregnant women (*see* pp. 35–36). There are, however, some important exceptions.

• *Watch your intake of vitamin B_6.* With so many apparently healthy people being deficient in vitamin B_6,[4] probably because of exposure to herbicides and other environmental B_6 antagonists (pp. 10, 33), it is perhaps not surprising that breastfeeding mothers must supplement their diets with 20 mg a day of vitamin B_6 just to make sure their infants receive the R D A of this vitamin.[5] On the other hand, excess vitamin B_6 (at levels of 200 mg a day or more) can inhibit lactation (i.e. milk production). If you have difficulty producing enough milk, cut the vitamin B_6 you take back to 10 mg a day.

• *Eliminate the manganese supplement.* During your baby's first four-to-six weeks, her brain is exceptionally susceptible to the toxic effects of this mineral. Excess manganese is suspected of contributing to the later development of hyperactivity in youngsters. (*See also* the data on high manganese formulas, p. 53.)

The amounts of most other vitamins and minerals in breast milk will not increase above normal levels even if you take large amounts as supplements. These include vitamins C, K and B_3 (nicotinic acid), folic acid and biotin, and the minerals sodium, calcium, zinc, fluorine, copper and iron. Taking these in supplements will build up your own body's stores, but will not affect your baby.

If you take in enough iron during pregnancy, your baby will be born with enough in her bone marrow and liver to be in good health. But you should be aware that, by the time your breastfed child is nine or ten months old, these stores of iron may be used up. Luckily, by that time most babies are ready for foods that contain iron.

WHAT *NOT* TO TAKE WHILE BREASTFEEDING

The last thing you will want to do is to transmit any toxins (poisons) to your baby through your breast milk. Consult your doctor before taking any drugs while breastfeeding. In particular, avoid every item on the following short list of drugs, drinks, additives and other substances.

DRUGS

• *Opiates* (including cough syrups with codeine). If you *must* take such medications, be sure *not* to nurse your infant for at least *four hours* afterwards.

• *Tranquillizers,* whether *barbiturates* or *benzodiazepines* such as Valium or Librium.

• *Aspirin* can interfere with your baby's normal blood-clotting activity – avoid it. If for some reason you *must* take it, don't breastfeed for *four hours* afterwards.

- *Paracetamol* can damage your infant's liver.
- *Cough syrups containing iodine* (in the form of potassium iodide) can affect your baby's thyroid function. You don't have to worry about the iodine in shellfish, though.
- *Caffeine* is actually a drug, because the body becomes addicted to it. It can cause irritability and sleeplessness in your infant as well as yourself.
- *Nicotine* is also a drug – don't smoke. The nicotine in cigarette tobacco can affect your baby's heartrate and produce vomiting and diarrhoea.
- *Alcohol*, even in small quantities, can damage your baby's brain cells. Drink fruit juice or soda water instead.
- *Illegal drugs* such as *marijuana* and *cocaine* can interfere with the functioning of your infant's developing brain.

FOOD/DRINK

Chocolate contains theobromine, easily transmitted in breast milk. It can make your infant irritable.

ADDITIVES

Aspartame, commercially called NutraSweet, can be toxic to newborns, making them hyperexcitable. Some experiments with animals suggest that it may cause brain damage as well.

ENVIRONMENTAL POLLUTANTS

Pesticides are fat soluble and therefore easily transmitted in breast milk. (They enter your milk before being stored in your own body fat.) Large amounts of PCB herbicides (such as Agent Orange) have been identified in the milk of young mothers in many countries. What can you do? First, avoid obvious large pesticide exposures. Don't arrange to have pests exterminated or your lawn fertilized (fertilizers often contain weed- and bug-killers). Stay away from the countryside when landowners are spraying crops.

Second, do not diet while breastfeeding. The pesticides and herbicides that you have unknowingly consumed and inhaled for most of your life are stored in your body's fat tissue, where they are relatively harmless. Stringent diets that promote brisk weight loss release these stored toxins into your blood, increasing their concentration in your milk. When nursing your baby, you should eat heartily, not only to ensure good nutritional quality for your milk, but to keep pesticides out.

When Should You Not Breastfeed?

There are two conditions under which breastfeeding can be harmful to your baby. If you are taking drugs to treat a disease, check with your doctor about their potential toxicity for your infant. If your baby has a disease, ask your doctor whether breastfeeding might adversely affect her. The commonest condition that can be made worse by breast milk is a jaundice of the newborn. Jaundice is a yellow discolouration of skin and eyes caused by the accumulation of a natural chemical called bilirubin in the blood. Normally, the liver excretes bilirubin into the bile, but in many newborns, the liver is unable to do this efficiently at the time of birth. In older infants and children, bilirubin itself is non-toxic, although jaundice may be a sign of serious disease. In newborns, jaundice is not usually a sign of disease, just of age, but bilirubin can be toxic to the brain if high enough blood levels are reached. Breast milk contains substances that can slow the excretion of bilirubin by the liver. If your newborn infant has serious jaundice, such that hospitalization or medical therapy is being contemplated, see if a temporary cessation of breastfeeding (one to two weeks should be enough) allows the condition to improve.[6]

HOW TO MANAGE BREASTFEEDING AND WORK

How do you breastfeed fulltime and still hold down a job? It's not easy, but it can be done. There are three possible options:

• *Do both at once.* This is the hardest one. If you are lucky enough to have the kind of work situation that permits it, you can bring your baby to work with you and breastfeed there. But even if your co-workers are enormously supportive, it can be exhausting to try to give 100 per cent to both your baby and your job.

• *Adjust your job to your baby's needs.* This is a popular solution, but it's not always possible. It depends on the kind of work you do. By working part-time, or sharing a job with someone else, though, you can breastfeed fulltime without sacrificing the energy you need for your job and your baby.

• *Adjust your baby's nursing to your fulltime job.* This is the most prevalent solution, but it means that you will have to express your milk into sterile containers and refrigerate or freeze it. Your care giver can then bottle-feed your breast milk to your baby while you are at work.

The catch is that most women can express only a few ounces of milk at a time, whereas a baby needs 4 fluid ounces per feeding. This means you will have to express milk several times to accumulate enough for a baby's needs while you are at work.

A SCHEDULE FOR BREASTFEEDING WHEN YOU WORK FULLTIME

This has worked for many mothers.

Morning. Get up about an hour earlier than you normally do. This gives you 15 minutes for your own needs. Use the next 45 minutes in these segments:

    10 minutes to breastfeed on one side.
    10 minutes to wind (not usually necessary) and hold your baby.
    10 minutes to breastfeed the other side.
    15 minutes to gently pat, wind and cradle your baby to sleep (you hope).

Lunchtime. Breastfeeding during the day is only practical if you live near your work. You can go home to breastfeed at lunchtime or, if you have the option, have your care giver bring the baby to you at work for breastfeeding in your private office or a comfortable corner of the women's lounge, assuming you have the former or the latter exists, and you can arrange the time. If you nurse in your private office, you may find that co-workers who barge in on you are nonplussed at first. One mother hangs a sign on her door to warn colleagues to wait a few minutes.

If you don't live close enough to work to make breastfeeding practical, your care giver will give your baby a warmed bottle of refrigerated or frozen breast milk.

After Work. Tell your care giver what time you expect to get home so that he or she won't feed your baby for at least an hour before you arrive. That way, you can feed your baby as soon as you get home. If you expect to be delayed, ask the care giver to feed the baby some cooled-down (warm to the touch) boiled water.

You may find it helpful to breastfeed your baby two or three times after you arrive home, including, if you wish, once just before bed. This helps her to feel full and sleepy by the time you are ready for bed yourself.

When Can You Express Your Milk?

Most women can express a fluid ounce of milk in about five minutes, and in an average feeding, babies will take in about 4 fluid ounces. If you have enough milk, you can express some milk just before feeding your baby in the morning and evening. You can also express enough milk over a weekend for your baby to drink while you are at work during the week. If you can arrange the privacy, you can express milk during the workday, but only if you can refrigerate it until you get home. (In fact, when you breastfeed, your breasts will tend to fill with milk every two hours, so you will feel more comfortable if you can express milk or nurse during the day.) You can express your milk either manually or with a breast pump. Both the National Childbirth Trust and the La Lèche League can teach you how to do this.

Breast milk is highly perishable; refrigerate or freeze it in sterile containers. (Plastic bags shouldn't be used because substances in the plastic that keep it soft can dissolve in the fat of the milk and will be consumed by your infant. These plastic softeners have been shown to cause cancer in experimental animals.) Sterilize heat-proof glass jars by boiling them in water for 20 minutes. Let them cool from hot to warm, then fill with breast milk and refrigerate or freeze. Refrigerated breast milk will keep for 24 hours; frozen, it will keep for up to 30 days.

You can add fresh breast milk to a partially filled container of frozen milk and return the container to the freezer, but only if you add less than the amount already frozen. If you add more, the fresh warm milk will thaw the frozen, and this may change its quality and allow bacteria to grow.

BOTTLE-FEEDING

If it's not possible to breastfeed fulltime with any of the arrangements above, it's still better to breastfeed part-time than not at all. And that means your care giver will feed your child a formula while you're at work. *If at all possible, though, do try to breastfeed fulltime for her first six weeks of life.* There are no perfect formulas for very young infants, either in terms of nutrition or of immune protection. Infants under six weeks are especially susceptible to infections; they need the protection breast milk provides.

Infant formulas are all contaminated with aluminium, a toxic metal, and contain 30 to 100 times as much aluminium as breast milk.[7] In infants with kidney disease, formula feeding can cause brain damage from aluminium toxicity. The effect of aluminium on normal newborns is not known.

If you are unable to breastfeed at all, you will have to supplement your baby's formula to compensate for its lack of EFAs and anti-oxidants. After I've discussed formulas, I will provide detailed information on how to supplement them.

Cow's or goat's milk?

I don't believe children should have cow's milk until they're a year old. Many infants are allergic to it because their digestive tracts haven't developed enough to be able to handle it. Studies show that the overabundance of the protein *casein* in cow's milk can curdle. The result? Your baby feels discomfort and spits up the milk.

Goat's milk is a fair *occasional* substitute for breast milk, but it's too low in folic acid and vitamin B_{12} to be adequate as your child's sole food; in addition, it contains a relatively high level of sodium. While it's not as overrich in protein as cow's milk, it still has much more than human breast milk, and must be diluted two to one with water. Since, unlike breast milk, it isn't sterile, it has to be boiled.

Milk-based formulas

Although they have their drawbacks, milk-based formulas are the best and most convenient substitutes for breast milk. Processing renders their protein less allergenic, but look for a formula that lists added whey. Whey and casein are different components of milk. Casein is harder to digest and more allergenic than whey, and, as I pointed out above, cow's milk contains more casein than human milk. Added whey means that the ratio of whey and casein in the formula has been adjusted to approximate that of breast milk.

A high manganese content is a serious problem with some formulas, because newborns may be particularly susceptible to the toxic effects of excess manganese. Many learning-disabled children have higher than normal amounts of manganese in their hair, and although we don't know whether the cause is excessive absorption of manganese or too much manganese in food, the problem may start in the first few months of life.[8]

For the first three months, a formula should be low in iron, too, to avoid the risk of gastro-enteritis. (*See* p. 43 for a discussion of the problems infants have with iron.) In fact, for the first four months, look for a formula that's low in both manganese and iron. After that, switch to one that is iron-fortified. Note that when you sterilize a formula, you inevitably destroy some of the added vitamins, among them C and B_6 (pyridoxine).

Soya formulas

I don't recommend any of these because they are low in *carnitine*, a substance essential for proper fat metabolism. They are useful for children who are allergic to cow's milk formulas, while providing approximately the same nutrition. But they contain up to nine times more manganese than breast milk.

SOME TIPS ON FORMULA FEEDING

● *Check the lead content of your water supply.* Ask your water board for the statistics, or have your water checked by a private laboratory. (Try running the

cold water for three or more minutes in the morning to flush out any lead
leached in overnight from soldering on pipe joints.) If it has a lead content
greater than 0.03 parts per million, use a ready-to-feed formula that doesn't
require added water, or use bottled spring water in preparing formula.

• *If you use tap water, boil it uncovered for five minutes before adding it to the
formula.* This will kill germs and help evaporate the chlorine added to all tap
water.

• *Never, ever, give a bottle to a sleepy or sleeping child.* While she may feed in her
sleep by reflex, problems are likely. At worst, she can choke.

COMPENSATING FOR A FORMULA'S NUTRITIONAL DEFICITS

All formulas are inadequate in GLA and omega-3 EFA, and some contain
no added taurine. If you breastfeed part-time, and you are well nourished,
your milk will compensate for these inadequacies. If you can't breastfeed at
all, you should supplement the formula. Fortunately, this isn't hard to do.

GLA

One good source is Efamol (brand) evening primrose oil. It comes in 500-mg
capsules. Another source is blackcurrant seed oil, which comes in either 250-
or 500-mg capsules. Once a day, rub the oil from one 250-mg capsule of
either oil into your baby's skin (the inner thigh and the inner forearm are the
best places). It will be absorbed into her body. (*See* p. 15 for a complete
discussion of evening primrose oil and other sources of EFAs.) *Under no
circumstances should you try to get a child under four years old to swallow a capsule.*

Omega-3 EFA

The best source is organically grown, food-grade linseed oil, found in
healthfood shops. Your baby can take a total of 1 teaspoon (5 ml) a day in her
formula, divided among three feedings. Add one-third of this measure to a
bottle before sterilization. If your baby has no problem with it, try adding the
whole measure at once. If linseed oil is not available, use four drops of cod-
liver oil or ⅓ tablespoon (5 ml) of walnut oil three times a day. Oils contain no
protein, so they are not major allergens. (*See* p. 13 for a complete discussion
of linseed oil and other sources of EFAs.)

You can also rub linseed or walnut oil into her skin. In India, infants are
regularly anointed with oil as part of a ritual of love and tenderness. One
teaspoonful (5 ml) of linseed or walnut oil will anoint your infant's entire
body. Don't use more than that. The skin will absorb the oil on its own; you
don't need to rub it all in.

Two important warnings about linseed oil:
- *It should have almost no taste. If it tastes even slightly bitter, it is rancid; throw it out.*
- *Never use artists' linseed oil. It is poison. Use only the food-grade varieties.*

HOW TO HANDLE FEEDING PROBLEMS

I can't tell whether my child is irritable, hungry or sick. Does every cry mean I should feed my baby?

A whimper doesn't mean distress or hunger – you don't have to nurse your baby continually. A sudden strong cry or wail usually means your infant is uncomfortable, but a small tired cry may just mean some temporary irritation. If you think your child is out of sorts but not hungry, try changing her nappy, or even just talking or singing to her in a quiet, soothing voice.

Life is made harder for working mothers by the fact that most children get fussy and need attention around 6.00 P.M. So if you are rushing home from work every night to be with your child, you will be asked to drop your own needs the minute you arrive – even though that's just when you need some quiet moments yourself.

Drs Urs Hunziker and Ronald Barr of Montreal Children's Hospital in Canada found that infant-carrying practices play a large role in determining the irritability of young infants and may account for the greater frequency of crying among babies in industrial countries than that found in traditional, pre-industrial cultures. In industrial societies, a crying infant can become an incessant problem for some parents, eroding coping skills and possibly contributing to child abuse. Crying tends to peak about the sixth week. In a study that compared the effect of extra carrying with other forms of attention, Drs Hunziker and Barr found that two hours a day of extra carrying during the first three months of life produced a 43 per cent decrease in crying and fussing, increased 'awake contentment' as reported by the mothers, and eliminated the six-week crying peak. A baby sling or back carrier is a handy way to accomplish this, and can be used by your partner and care giver as well. Not only will you increase 'carrying time', you will also increase physical contact with your baby and become more attuned to her moods and movements. If carrying the baby hurts your back, look for one that carries your baby on your hip.

Your child's colour and temperature will tell you whether she is really sick. As long as she's pink, she's probably fine. If she turns blue, grey or blotchy, she's probably ill. Suddenly cold hands and feet may indicate a problem, too.

Here are some other signals to look for:

- *Signs of mild dehydration.* Are her eyes and mouth dry? Does her skin seem dry and less elastic than when she is well?
- *A lack of responsiveness.* Does she fail to respond to your smiles, gestures and cuddling? Does she seem bored with her toys?
- *A different kind of cry.* Her crying may sound angrier, more intense, more distraught.
- *Excessive sleepiness.* Is she sleeping more than usual? Do you have a hard time waking her up?
- *Glassy eyes.* Just as you do when you have a cold or flu, your infant may become glassy-eyed when she is sick.

What do I do if she is sick and doesn't want to eat?
When your infant is sick, she will need less food than usual; never force food on her. But if she seems dehydrated (*see above*), give her water to drink. If she has a cold and is dripping mucus, you can use a nasal saltwater wash to dissolve it. Add ⅛ teaspoon of table salt or coarse salt to half a glass (about 4 fluid ounces/115 ml) of boiled, cooled water. Use the tip of a nose or ear dropper to squirt this solution *into the edge* of (not up) the nostril. If you haven't a dropper, dip a clean, soft cotton handkerchief into the salt water, wring it out and gently wipe away the mucus.

What if I have a cold or sore throat? Should I stop breastfeeding and keep away from my baby?
No! Keep right on breastfeeding – just take some precautions. Wash your hands carefully before you go near the baby, and if you like, you can wear a respiratory mask or a handkerchief when you hold her. However, since you incubate a cold for some time before showing any symptoms, it is likely that your baby will have already caught yours.

If you have a cold, take a lot of fluids – water, orange juice, hot chicken soup, herbal teas. And this is the time for megadoses of vitamin C: 1000 to 3000 mg every hour. If you get a touch of diarrhoea, you will know you have reached your limit of tolerance and you can lower your dosage. These megadoses won't get into your breast milk, so you don't have to worry about affecting your baby.

For a sore throat, I always find it helpful to keep my throat warm and to gargle with salt water. Zinc lozenges (no more than five a day) can relieve pain. Hot lemon drinks made with fresh lemon juice and a touch of honey are an old and effective remedy. As with a cold, drink lots of liquids and take megadoses of vitamin C.

If my baby has colic, could my diet be responsible?
I've long thought that colic in breastfed babies might have something to do with the mother's consumption of cow's milk. Swedish doctors studied 18 mothers of colicky babies who eliminated milk from their diets. In 13 of the babies, the colic disappeared.

Also watch for hard-to-digest foods or drinks, as these are apt to be passed along to the baby in breast milk. Avoid such 'wind'-producing foods as beans, lentils, Brussels sprouts, broccoli, cabbage, mushrooms, fizzy drinks, and, of course, alcohol. Also watch spices! Recently, a young mother told me of how she had gleefully gone out for her first restaurant meal after her baby's birth. 'We went to a wonderful Mexican restaurant,' she told me. 'I certainly learned a lot about spices! Paavo was sick and irritable for the next 24 hours!'

My baby seems too hungry for the amounts of milk my breasts can supply – or she doesn't seem to grow well on breast milk alone.
Remember, infants are hungry frequently – in fact, it's natural for everyone, adults as well as infants, to want to feed every 90 minutes. Three meals a day is simply a convention that allows society to get its work done. So if your baby is hungry often, that doesn't necessarily mean your milk is inadequate. If she isn't growing as fast as she should, your doctor or health visitor may advise you to supplement your own milk with a formula. But as long as breastfeeding remains her major source of nourishment, she will still benefit from all the special nutrients in your milk.

Unfortunately, there is no magic formula for increasing the amount of milk you are able to supply. You will produce more if you are relaxed and calm, if you eat about 1900 calories a day, breastfeed frequently, and watch your intake of vitamin B_6 (pyridoxine), for that could interfere with lactation. Don't take more than 30 mg of vitamin B_6 a day. If you are breastfeeding part-time, you will probably keep up a better flow of milk if you breastfeed at night rather than giving your baby a bottle.

How will I know when it's time to wean my baby?
There is no 'right age' for weaning a baby. Ideally, your baby will wean herself completely, sometime after 11 months. As she learns to love solid foods, she will feed less frequently at your breast. You can encourage her to wean herself by feeding her solid foods more frequently, which brings us to the question of how to introduce your baby to solid foods.

Six Months to a Year:
Building Up Young Bodies
When Starting Solid Food

4

At some point between his fourth and seventh month, a baby is ready to start eating solid food. Don't rush this moment; for both your sakes, it's better for him to start solid food later rather than earlier. The best thing to do is to let him tell you when he's ready: he will be able to sit up well and he will seem hungrier than usual between his feeds. A sure sign is that he will begin moving his tongue back and forth in his mouth, rather than up and down in the sucking pattern. This means he is ready to move food from his lips to his throat.

There are some very good reasons not to rush your baby into solid food:
• When he starts eating solid foods, the wonderfully protective *Lactobacillus bifidus* will disappear from his intestinal tract. At seven months, he will be better able to handle this loss than at four months.
• Assuming you've been breastfeeding, the extra couple of months of breast milk will help sustain and enhance his developing immune system, minimizing any chance of food allergies.[1] Allergenic reactions will increase the susceptibility of his intestinal and respiratory tracts to infection, just at the point when he is susceptible anyway because he is losing his *bifidus* protection.
• It's much more convenient for you, because at seven months he can handle mashed food; you won't have to purée or strain everything.

On the other hand, I don't see any reason to prolong exclusive breastfeeding much past seven months. A century ago, babies were given no solids until they were a year old, which wasn't a bad idea at the time. Hygiene was relatively poor and the incidence of intestinal-tract infections was high. But my experience is that babies are physiologically ready for solid foods at seven months.

At that age, the limitations of breast milk start to become significant, too. It is low in iron and vitamin D, and may not provide enough calories or protein for an older baby's growth. So, although I advocate nothing but breast milk for the first six months, at seven months it is definitely time for solid food.

Here are some common questions mothers often ask me about this transition:
Can you prevent food allergies if you breastfeed exclusively for a full year?
Unfortunately, breast milk only delays the onset of food allergies; it can't prevent them altogether. Good nutrition, with special attention to EFAs, will do a good deal more to prevent allergies than delaying solid foods.

How can you tell if you've started solid foods too soon?
If he spits them out, or drools when he's fed, he's probably not ready; wait a few more weeks. Don't try to force him to eat; stop feeding as soon as he stops eating.

What if he resists spoon feeding?
Many babies go through this stage, either because they want to keep sucking or because they want to feed themselves. Don't force-feed your baby; it will just build frustration and increase resistance. I don't advise adding sugar to food either; that will just accustom him to overly sweet foods and contribute to tooth decay. If he wants to suck, let him breastfeed longer. When he gets hungry enough so that breast milk no longer suffices, he will start to accept solids.

If he doesn't want to let you put the spoon into his mouth, and grasps at the spoon or the food – or both – you'll know he wants to feed himself. If he's able to grasp with his fingers, he may be ready to feed himself at least some of the time. But if he grasps with his palm, he's not ready.

What should you do? Give him thick, sticky food that he can grasp with his palm and put into his mouth: big lumps of thick, cold baby cereal or moistened, fork-mashed potatoes; mashed vegetables stuck together with oatmeal; or pieces of peeled soft fruit. This kind of food gives him a more varied diet than milk alone, and helps him develop the pincer grasp that will enable him to hold a spoon.

At first he will play with his food more than he'll eat it. But if he eats with his parents or siblings, their example and his own hunger should have him eating more and playing less before your patience runs out.

INTRODUCING YOUR BABY TO SOLID FOODS

HOW TO START

Until now, your baby has had nothing but liquids with a fairly limited range of taste. Now he is ready for cereal, fruits and vegetables (high-protein foods come later). You won't want to overwhelm him with new tastes and textures. A good rule of thumb is to introduce new foods one at a time.

Giving him a larger amount of a single food at a feeding, rather than small amounts of several foods, allows him to get used to a new food so that he'll be less likely to reject it. He'll also be less likely to have an allergic reaction. Strange as it seems, a small amount of a new food is more likely to induce a baby's immune system to form allergic antibodies than is a larger amount.

You will want to start your baby on soft, bland, smooth foods, such as cereal. Then, over a period of four to six months, he can learn to accept different tastes and textures while he develops chewing skills and learns to feed himself. When he's mastered cereal, you can add foods with a coarser texture and stronger taste. Cooking and puréeing will make even such vegetables as beans suitable until he is ready for chunky, chewy foods such as broccoli. Last of all come finger foods such as cooked carrot sticks. By this time, your baby will be ready to start eating his meals at the table with the rest of the family. (But it's not necessary to worry about what he eats at what time of day. At this point, it's all just food to him.)

Food No. 1: Iron-Fortified Cereal

You will want to start your baby off on iron-fortified rice, oat or barley cereal. No wheat until he's a year old, because it's more likely to produce an allergic reaction.

The iron is important because, by this time, your child's iron stores are used up, and he needs more so that his brain will develop properly. Studies have shown that children who are only mildly iron-deficient – so mildly that they aren't anaemic – score lower on tests of mental function than children that aren't lacking in this important mineral. Correcting the iron deficiency improves mental performance.[2]

Iron will also prevent anaemia and enable his body to resist infection. Contrary to the belief of certain people, an iron deficiency at this age will not protect a baby against infection. In fact, it can only do him harm. As we saw in the last chapter, it is only newborn infants who have problems with iron. (Older children and adults with *serious* protein deficiencies are unable to use iron either, but that is another story.)

Furthermore, iron deficiency increases the absorption of lead from food.[3]

Increases in the blood lead level, even within the so-called 'safe' range, adversely affects the intellectual function and academic achievement of children.⁴ Lead enters food through processing (lead solder in cans) and from house dust.⁵

Preparing your baby's cereal. Use breast milk or formula as the liquid. You will want to start with a consistency only slightly thicker than milk. As your child becomes able to handle it, you can gradually thicken it to the more usual consistency. A good method is to start with a thin cereal broth and gradually add more cereal to get the texture you want. Feed a very small amount – about ⅛ teaspoon – at a time, slowly increasing the amount as he grows accustomed to it.

Every three days or so, he should be ready for a new cereal. A good order is a rice cereal, then oatmeal, then a barley cereal. If you use a dry cereal, you will, of course, soak it thoroughly until it is soft, then dilute it to the right consistency.

Food No. 2: Vegetables

Once your baby is happily eating cereals, he's ready to meet vegetables. Start with puréed green beans and peas, marrows and potatoes.

Don't give your baby spinach, beetroot, turnips, carrots or greens until he is nine months old. While they are excellent sources of important nutrients, especially vitamin A, these vegetables may be too rich in nitrates for him before then. Nitrates can change his red blood cells so that they are less able to carry oxygen.

Food No. 3: Fruit

About a month after starting vegetables, he should be ready to tackle fruit. I recommend apples (puréed), peaches, apricots, pears, nectarines and plums. Avoid bananas – their porous skin admits the toxic fungicides that are sprayed on imported fruits. (In general, avoid any imported fruits, but bananas are the most dangerous. They are not so problematic for older children, but infants' immature livers are ill-prepared to detoxify and eliminate pesticides. Older, heavier children, whose livers function better, will not be harmed by the occasional piece of imported fruit.) To be on the safe side, *use only washed or peeled local fruits in season*. Out-of-season fruit may well be imported. Buy ripened fruits – they're tastiest and most nutritious, and are the easiest to mash or purée.

Start with cooked fruit; it's easiest to bake it. Preheat the oven to 350°F/180C/gas mark 4. Wash the fruit. To preserve its nutrients, bake it in its skin in a covered dish with just a little water. When it's tender, it's done.

You can also steam it in a tightly covered pot. Either way, peel before puréeing or mashing. You probably won't have to add water for a smooth purée, since both cooking methods preserve natural liquids as well as nutrients. If you must add water, use the absolute minimum.

When your child can handle cooked fruit, try uncooked mashed fruit. The chewier texture will help him learn to chew. If he has a good grasp and can chew, you can give him small pieces to hold, chew and suck on. *Caution:* he must be able to chew well, mashing the fruit on his own, or he might choke on hard fruit, such as apple or pear.

Food No. 4: More Vegetables

Once he's mastered fruits, your baby is ready for chewier vegetables: courgette, broccoli, cauliflower, asparagus tips, kale and tomatoes. (Although they are soft and easily puréed, he won't be ready for tomatoes any earlier because of their acidity and strong taste.)

He's also old enough now to eat spinach, beetroot, turnips, carrots and greens. Serve each one every four to five days until he becomes familiar with them. Don't make the servings too large. If he shows 'windiness' or bloating, especially after eating turnips or greens, wait about a month before trying them again.

TIPS ON FOOD PREPARATION

● *It's best to prepare your baby's food yourself.* These days, with a blender or food processor, or both, in almost every home, it's easy to purée fresh vegetables. It's also simple to strain them. Either way is fine.

● *Leave out sugar, salt and fat.* These anti-nutrients do nothing for your baby, and, as we saw in Chapter 1, they slow down EFA metabolism. And *that* distorts the production line of prostaglandins, the chemicals that keep the immune system running properly. Anti-nutrients also increase the body's need for certain nutrients: sugar demands more B vitamins for its metabolism, while salt increases the amount of magnesium lost in the urine.

Babies love sweet foods, but they can get all the sweetness they want from fruits. If you add sugar, you're just adding empty calories while discouraging your child from acquiring more subtle tastes.

Never give honey to a child who is less than a year old. It could be contaminated with spores from botulism-causing bacteria. The Centers for Disease Control, the US national disease clearinghouse in Atlanta, Georgia, has reported infant deaths from botulism poisoning because of contaminated honey.

The desire for added salt is an acquired taste. Your baby won't think unsalted foods are bland; to him, they'll be interesting new tastes.

Commercial baby foods

There are some good-quality commercial products on the market, but be sure to check the labels to see that they don't contain additives of any sort – don't buy any that list sugar, salt, BHT (E321) or BHA (E320) – preservatives that may be allergenic or toxic – or EDTA, a colour-preserving agent that binds to minerals such as calcium and magnesium, preventing their absorption. EDTA, sugar and salt are all anti-nutrients.

Years ago, baby-food manufacturers routinely added sugar and salt to please a mother's taste buds. Today, though, some major producers offer natural baby foods, free of sugar, salt and preservatives. These products are sterile and nutritionally about as good as the food you prepare yourself. Note, though, that the chances are that any baby food labelled 'dessert' has been sweetened. In the US, H. J. Heinz has ordered the farmers producing crops for their baby foods to discontinue using 12 (legal) chemicals as pesticides.

Buy food in jars, not tins – canned baby foods may be contaminated by the lead used to solder the seams. Choose 'single' foods rather than 'dinners' combining different foods. In addition to consisting of more than one food, the dinners are more likely to contain added fat and salt.

TEN MONTHS: PROTEIN TIME

Until now, your infant's kidneys and digestive tract were not ready to handle high-protein foods. But these foods are rich in vitamins and minerals, too, and your baby is finally ready to take advantage of them.

At this point, he will be getting most of his nutrition from solid foods. He is ready for meat, poultry, beans, egg yolks (save the whites for another couple of months; they can be allergenic at this stage) and tofu (bean curd). This last, an easy-to-use form of the highly nutritious soyabean, is found in many shops today.

Beans work best when combined with grains to produce a more complete protein. Many cultures around the world have evolved staple dishes of this combination: rice and beans in Latin America; maize and lima beans, known in the US as 'succotash', sesame seeds and chickpeas in the Middle East. For a baby, make hummus – sesame butter (tahini) and ground chickpeas.

Seeds and nuts are also rich in proteins, vitamins and minerals – and EFAs as well. Nut butters are easy to make and your infant will enjoy them now and throughout his childhood (*see* p. 216 for the recipe). If you like, you can purée meat and poultry from your table for him. Skip fish, though, until he is a year old. Like egg whites, they are likely to be allergenic.

Finger-lickin' good. One of the many nice things about being ten months old is enjoying real finger foods. Give him pieces of fresh peeled fruit (with cores, stones, etc. removed), tofu chunks or small pieces of moist cooked chicken. (These are bigger, chewier foods than the small, soft pieces of fruit you may have given him earlier.)

EFAs. To be sure your baby is getting enough of the all-important omega-3 EFAs, it's a good idea to add about 1 teaspoon (5 ml) of food-grade linseed oil or 1 tablespon (15 ml) of walnut oil to his meals each day. You can mix it into meat and vegetable dishes. Taste linseed oil before using it. It should have virtually no taste, although some people detect a very slight fishy aftertaste. If it tastes bitter, it is rancid; throw it out.

ONE YEAR OLD: THE OMNIVOROUS EATER

At this age, your baby can eat almost anything. He has a few teeth, so he can chew more, and his digestive system can handle whole milk, whole eggs, yoghurt, fish and wheat. He will want to feed himself, and you should encourage him to do so as much as possible. You will still have to cut up his food, but he can pick the pieces with his hands and put them in his mouth. He may miss occasionally, but he'll learn. By this time, he should be eating at the table with the rest of the family.

In his new-found joy of eating, there is one danger: food that can slip down his windpipe. He's not really ready yet for whole nuts, raw carrots (the small chunks he bites off can create trouble) or popcorn. These won't be safe for him to eat until he is about 18 months old.

Serving Suggestions   You can crumble wholewheat toast into very small pieces and soak it in milk. You can also purée cooked wholewheat pasta in a small amount of milk.

Mash fish after removing both skin and bones.

At this stage of life, give your baby plain, whole-milk yoghurt rather than cow's milk. Yoghurt is more digestible, and adds beneficial lactobacillus organisms to his intestinal tract. You can mix fresh fruit with it, but stay away from the commercial high-sugar, yoghurt-with-fruit combinations. Many of these contain preservatives, as well. Your child will enjoy plain yoghurt all his life if he acquires a taste for it now.

DOES YOUR CHILD NEED SUPPLEMENTS?

You may already be giving your baby multivitamin drops and possibly fluoride drops as well. However, I don't believe that a healthy infant who is eating well needs any supplement except linseed oil, and I have serious reservations about the use of fluorides (see the section on tooth care that follows this one). Nevertheless, such supplements are probably harmless.

If your child is prone to infections, he will need more than the average multivitamin. Give him the following every day:

Vitamin C	200 mg
Folic acid	400 micrograms (0.04 mg)
Iron	10 mg
Zinc	5 mg

Vitamin D is actually not a vitamin at all – it's a hormone formed in the body by the action of sunlight. There is very little vitamin D in breast milk or cow's milk, although the latter is usually vitamin-D fortified. But the best source of vitamin D is still sunlight. It doesn't take much; 15 minutes a day at midday, summer or winter, even fully clothed, is enough. The sun on his hands and face will do the job. In the early morning or late afternoon, double the time. In southern climes, he will need less time; in the northern ones, a bit more.

Children whose skin is dark, or those who live in the far north, may have a problem getting enough sun during the winter. They can take 100 mg of infant vitamin D every day. Older children shouldn't need a supplement because so many commercial foods (including meat) have been directly or indirectly fortified with vitamin D (animal feed is laced with it).

HOW TO START THE TEETH OFF RIGHT

Tooth decay is endemic in children today, but you can do a lot to prevent it. Even before you can see your baby's teeth, they are right under the skin of his gums, and sugar, the worst culprit in tooth decay, can already begin to affect them. And even though you are keeping refined sugar, honey and treacle out of his diet altogether, you still have to deal with the natural sugars in fruits and root vegetables. A few rules of thumb will help:

● *Never give your baby fruit juice in a bottle.* Wait until he can drink from a cup. When he sucks from a bottle, he bathes his mouth in sugar-laden fluids; when he drinks from a cup, the fluids leave his mouth more quickly.

● *Don't give him anything sweet before bedtime.* This includes fresh or dried fruit (preferably without added preservatives) or juice. During the day, his saliva continually washes his teeth and gums, carrying away sugars. But during sleep the saliva flow is much reduced, so sugars stay longer in the mouth.

What about fluorides?

Fluoride, whether occurring naturally in water or added as a supplement, can strengthen teeth against decay. But *too much* can inhibit the action of certain enzymes in your baby's blood as well as causing brown strains on his teeth. Tooth decay is caused by an excess of sugar, not a deficiency of fluoride; there is no evidence that fluoride supplements help prevent decay if taken beyond the first year of life.

THE 'INVISIBLE' NUTRIENT

When you breastfed your baby, the two of you were close, both physically and emotionally, and the bond between you steadily deepened. As he was weaned, you still spent a lot of time with him, feeding him and touching him, and he was still very dependent on you.

Now that he is beginning to be more independent, there will be progressively fewer occasions when you must touch him to care for him. As he grows older, he will do more and more things for himself, but you will want to keep the warm love you have built strong and alive while he begins to build ties with family and friends. Meals are good occasions for building and reinforcing these bonds; keep them easy, relaxed and happy.

COPING WITH HEALTH PROBLEMS

You can expect your baby to have minor problems during his first year of life – a cold or two, transient diarrhoea, equally transient irritability. But if he develops health problems that persist for longer than three weeks, they may signify an underlying disturbance. The most common chronic problems at this age are colic, diarrhoea, constipation, poor sleep, irritability, spitting up, congestion, coughs, nappy rash, recurrent throat and ear infections, and eczema (dermatitis).

In my experience, these problems usually occur against a background of food allergies and certain nutritional deficiencies. The most common deficiencies involve magnesium and EFAs. In addition, a child with recurrent infections may have a zinc, iron or vitamin A deficiency. If you follow my diet plan, your baby shouldn't have any dietary deficiencies, but some infants have trouble absorbing certain nutrients, or converting them to an active form.

In addition, a yeast – *Candida albicans* – can cause both severe nappy rash and thrush, a painful mouth infection. Infants are prone to *Candida* infections because their immune systems are immature. Antibiotics are often given to infants, sometimes inappropriately. These drugs kill normal bacteria in the intestine that prevent *Candida* from flourishing there. Once they are killed off, an overgrowth of yeast can lead to serious problems. *Candida* is a potent allergen, and *Candida*-induced allergies complicate the picture for many infants with chronic problems who have been given antibiotics.

Evaluating and treating any of these problems will involve one or more of the following:

- More EFAs
- More magnesium, sometimes with vitamins B_1 (thiamin) and B_6 (pyridoxine)
- For chronic infection, more iron, zinc and vitamin A
- A food-allergy evaluation
- Oral nystatin (an anti-fungal drug) and lactobacilli (the beneficial bacteria killed off by antibiotics, if a child has a yeast infection or a history of taking antibiotics)

In the pages that follow, I will take you step by step through the evaluation and treatment of these common chronic problems.

THE SYMPTOMS

Colic. He screams intensely, and he is not soothed by winding. He passes a great deal of wind and has abnormally hard or loose stools. He flexes his legs against his abdomen in an attempt to relieve the pain.

Diarrhoea. Loose or watery movements lasting more than a few days.

Constipation. Rock-hard, pebbly stool or bowel movements less often than every day.

Spitting up. He spits up even familiar foods.

Excess mucus, coughing or congestion. If any of these problems lasts more than three weeks, it is usually food-related.

Severe nappy rash. Persistent angry redness of the skin.

Recurrent throat and ear infections. See below, under Recurrent infections, page 74.

Eczema (dermatitis). Red, scaling patches of skin anywhere on the body.

Behavioural disturbances. Many temperamental children have been brought to me, usually after the age of one, by which time their problems have affected the whole family. Often these children are more alert, more inquisitive and brighter than other youngsters their age. They may even have reached certain developmental milestones earlier. But their poor adaptability and their negative moods can make them very hard to live with.

Dt Stanley Turecki of Mount Sinai Hospital in New York City has written an excellent book, *The Difficult Child* (1985), that lists some key traits that can be detected in an infant. In general, everything – people, touch, noises or music – seems to overstimulate him. He won't cuddle; when you try to hold him, he kicks and squirms a lot. Or he reacts to even gentle touching by withdrawing. It's hard to dress or bath him. He reacts to any unfamiliar noise as if it were a firecracker going off under his nose. He tends to be very loud himself, whether he is happy or sad. He is restless, fussy, cranky or irritable much of the time, and he sleeps irregularly and restlessly. He hates any change in routine. He eats on an irregular schedule, and reacts to new foods by spitting them out.

If any of these traits persist for over a month, you can consider them chronic.

THE MAGNESIUM CONNECTION IN COLIC AND BEHAVIOURAL PROBLEMS

The first step for young infants should be to increase 'carrying time' (*see above*, p. 55). If colic or temperamental behaviour become chronic, your baby might need magnesium supplementation, especially if he's over six months old. As I said above, if you are following my diet, your infant is unlikely to have a magnesium deficiency, but he might have trouble absorbing the mineral. This *creates* a deficiency that, in turn, affects calcium-regulating hormones. The result is a calcium deficiency. And that can cause intestinal spasms and irritability.

Babies with behavioural problems generally require more magnesium than do other infants – perhaps because the hormones secreted during their chronic high levels of stress trigger greater than normal excretion of magnesium in their urine.

In either case, 100 to 200 mg of magnesium a day should help. You will soon know if the dose is too high because excess magnesium causes diarrhoea. If that happens, simply cut back on the amount of magnesium, 50 mg at a time, until his stools are normal again.

Two inexpensive, easily available sources of magnesium are *magnesium citrate* and *milk of magnesia*: 100 mg of magnesium = ½ teaspoon (2.5 ml) magnesium citrate, or ½ teaspoon (2.5 ml) milk of magnesia. Add a tiny amount of either to your baby's food at each feeding, making sure the total reaches ½ to 1 teaspoon (2.5–5.0 ml) a day but does not exceed that amount. Magnesium generally has a calming effect and enhances sleep, a bonus in both colic and behavioural problems.

If magnesium supplements help with colic and/or sleep, or reduce irritability, I would continue them. The purest source for long-term use is magnesium citrate capsules. Magnesium citrate liquid and milk of magnesia often have artificial flavours and sweeteners added. However, magnesium citrate capsules are hard to find; if your local healthfood shop doesn't carry them, ask if they can order some for you.

Add B vitamins to aid magnesium absorption

The B vitamins, especially B_1 (thiamin) and B_6 (pyridoxine), help the body absorb and use magnesium more efficiently. If magnesium alone doesn't solve colic or behavioural problems, add 10 mg a day of *vitamin B_6 only* (B complex usually doesn't work as well) to your baby's diet. Your chemist may be able to make up a liquid form, free of additives.

If vitamin B_6 seems to have no effect, stop it and try 10 mg of B_1 a day, in the same liquid form.

Calcium for temperament

If magnesium alone doesn't seem to help your baby's behavioural problems, add calcium – 100 to 200 mg a day in the form of liquid calcium carbonate.

THE FOOD CONNECTION

Because many common problems start with food allergies, you may have to do a little nutritional detective work in the form of food trials to discover the food or foods that started the trouble. This should be your first step in dealing with diarrhoea and constipation, spitting up, coughing and congestion, and one form of severe nappy rash. For colic or behavioural problems, it is easier to try magnesium first; if that doesn't work, go on to a food trial.[6] For eczema (dermatitis), start with EFAs (*see below*), and then do a food trial.

The food trial

If you are breastfeeding, first check your own diet. For five days, stop taking all vitamins or drugs (be sure and check with your doctor before stopping any prescribed medication). Stop eating all possible allergenic foods: milk; wheat products; maize; soyabeans; eggs; caffeine; spices; green, orange or red vegetables; all fruit. Eat only such 'safe' foods as meat (lamb, beef, veal or pork), poultry, rice and potatoes. (These have all been statistically proved to be less allergenic.) If there is no change by the end of five days, the problem is not your diet; it's your baby's.

The most common allergen is cow's milk; if you are using a cow's milk formula, try changing to one based on soyabeans. (Casein in the milk could also be causing him to spit up.) If a soya formula doesn't stop the symptom, switch to a formula based on hydrolyzed vegetable protein.

If he is eating solid foods, cut him back to the safe foods, too: rice cereal, lamb, puréed apples. If he is taking vitamins, stop them altogether during this period. If his symptoms don't stop after five days, cut out the apples and feed him only lamb, rice and breast milk or hydrolyzed formula for five more days.

Once he stops showing symptoms, you can begin to add new foods carefully – one every two days. Feed each new food two or three times a day for two days. Watch carefully to see whether he develops any symptoms; if he does, cut the food out of his diet altogether and go on to the next. You can treat vitamins as you would a food, and add in one at a time.

Food allergy-caused nappy rash

What looks like nappy rash could be caused by food allergy. If so, the rash comes on suddenly and is bright red – the skin looks scalded. (Both these factors distinguish this rash from that caused by a yeast infection, described below.) Suspect a food eaten by one of you in the last 48 hours. It could take another 48 hours to clear up, depending on how quickly his body eliminates the toxic material. Because almost any food or additive could be the culprit, I suggest a food trial.

THE STRESS CONNECTION

You might also pay special attention to your own emotional state. Are you under stress? If you are emotionally upset, how do you react? By eating? By not eating? Do you become constipated? Whether or not you are breastfeeding, your behaviour and emotional state can trigger changes in your baby's behaviour – and that, in turn, can trigger more emotional stress in you.

THE EFA CONNECTION

Diarrhoea and constipation

Since both these conditions may be caused by an allergy, conduct a food trial first. If you don't discover the culprit, then you might suspect an EFA deficiency. (A diet too low in fats can cause diarrhoea, too.)

If your baby isn't getting linseed oil either directly or in your breast milk, add some to your diet or his. If he is getting linseed oil now, give him a larger dose: 1 tablespoon (15 ml) a day. (See p. 54 for suggestions on how to give linseed oil to a baby.) You may substitute 1 teaspoon (5 ml) of cod-liver oil or 2 tablespoons (30 ml) of walnut oil for 1 tablespoon (15 ml) of linseed oil.

Jeremy's family had a history of heart disease, which led his mother to give him no fats. He was eating solid foods and getting only skimmed milk when I first saw him at the age of ten months. He was suffering from loose bowel movements. I put him on whole milk and linseed oil, to provide both fats and EFAs. Jeremy's diarrhoea stopped, and his dry skin became smoother.

It is also worth noting that some vitamins – A, D, E and K – are fat-soluble and, therefore occur primarily in fats. Deficiency in these vitamins can occur if children under the age of five are kept on fat-restricted diets; giving whole milk is the easiest way of overcoming this.

Behavioural problems

When you've tried magnesium and, if necessary, done a food trial, it's time to look at EFAs. If your baby isn't getting linseed oil either directly or in your breast milk, add some to your diet or his. If he is getting linseed oil now, double the dose for you or for him. You may substitute walnut or cod-liver oil in the following ratios: 1 teaspoon (5 ml) of cod-liver oil for 1 tablespoon (15 ml) of linseed oil or 2 tablespoons (30 ml) of walnut oil for 1 tablespoon (15 ml) of linseed oil.

If you're not happy with the effects of linseed oil, apply two 250-mg capsules of evening primrose or blackcurrant seed oil directly on to his skin each day. (See p. 15 for detailed information on evening primrose oil and blackcurrant seed oil.)

I've seen these oils improve sleep and temperament within two days to two weeks. Take Jessie – at ten months, she was restless and difficult. It was impossible to hold and cuddle her; she would cry loudly until her face turned red, and she never slept more than two hours at a time. I first changed her from a milk- to soya-based formula. She stopped crying and passing wind, but she continued to be irritable and to sleep badly. Her parents wondered why she was thirsty all the time.

Excessive thirst suggested an EFA problem, but 2 teaspoons (10 ml) of linseed oil a day seemed to have no effect. I recommended two 250-mg capsules of evening primrose oil every day, rubbed into Jessie's skin. Within three days, she was no longer thirsty, and was sleeping longer and more soundly. But she was still restless and moved stiffly, so I recommended ¼ fluid ounce (approximately 7 ml, or just over 1 teaspoon) of liquid magnesium citrate a day. After two weeks, she was much calmer and moved more easily.

Persistent behavioural problems

If the food trials, magnesium and EFA supplementation outlined above don't result in significant improvement in your child's 'difficult' behaviour, and if he has most of the symptoms listed on page 67, it may be time to consult your doctor.

Eczema (dermatitis)

Some children need more EFAs than others because their bodies don't metabolize EFAs well. Children with eczema (medically known as *dermatitis*) have difficulty converting linoleic acid, the major omega-6 EFA, to GLA.[7] Evening primrose oil and blackcurrant seed oil, which contain GLA, get round this problem.

Such children may also need more omega-3 EFAs; up to 1 tablespoon (15 ml) of linseed oil a day by the age of one may help. Or you may substitute up to 1 teaspoon (5 ml) of cod-liver oil or up to 2 tablespoons (30 ml) of walnut oil. If you are breastfeeding, add EFAs to your own diet.

Food allergy usually complicates eczema, so a food trial of the kind outlined on pages 69–70 could help as well.[8]

At three months, Christopher had severe eczema. His mother, who breastfed him, was eating a lot of eggs. When she cut them out of her diet, Christopher's condition improved but didn't disappear entirely. To increase omega-3 EFAs in her milk, his mother added linseed and cod-liver oil to her diet. Over the next two months, Christopher's eczema cleared up and his dry skin improved.

Jennifer at nine months was skinny and a picky eater. Although she had dry skin and mild eczema, I didn't want to start eliminating foods from her diet because she was so thin. Instead, I advised rubbing two 250-mg primrose oil capsules and 1 teaspoon (5 ml) of linseed oil into her skin each day. Her eczema cleared up completely.

SEVERE NAPPY RASH: THE YEAST CONNECTION

Ordinary nappy rash – a light reddening of the skin – can be avoided. It's caused by urine and faeces, both of which irritate the skin. It can be prevented by frequent changes, gentle but thorough cleansing, powdering with corn-flour, and disposable nappies, especially in hot weather. If you are breast-feeding your child, he is less likely to get nappy rash, because breastmilk is more completely digested then formula, and as a result, his stools and urine contain fewer irritating substances.

Severe nappy rash – a persistent angry redness of the skin – is usually a symptom of a yeast infection. The yeast·Candida albicans thrives in a warm, dark, moist environment, so one step towards a cure is to let your baby go without a nappy as much as possible. Ointment containing vitamins A and D stimulates local immune response and is also soothing.

If none of these treatments works, doctors sometimes prescribe a cream containing a mixture of a steroid (to decrease inflammation), an antibiotic and nystatin (to kill yeast).

To prevent a yeast infection, your child should be helped to avoid unneeded antibiotics, whether he gets them through your milk or directly. Antibiotics are undiscriminating in the bacteria they kill off, and eliminate the useful bacteria that keep yeast infestations under control.

- If your baby is taking formula give him supplements of Lactobacillus bifidus.
- Keep sugar out of your diet and his, and take linseed oil: 1 teaspoon (5 ml) a day for him, 1 tablespoon (15 ml) a day for you.
- Provide a diet rich in zinc, iron and vitamin A. Egg yolks and liver are the best choice for your baby. Combine them with fruits with a high vitamin C content such as strawberries or oranges, or vegetables such as broccoli or tomatoes. Feed him one egg yolk or 2 ounces (55 g) of liver every day for two weeks, then reduce the amount to three egg yolks and 2 ounces (55 g) of liver a week. Don't give him more than that; with too much liver, you risk an overdose of vitamin A.
- Ask your doctor to prescribe an oral (by mouth) suspension of nystatin. This is the only prescription drug I advocate using aggressively with infants and young children. The widespread and generally excessive use of anti-biotics promotes intestinal Candida overgrowth, an important factor in the development of allergies. Commonly prescribed doses of nystatin – 100,000 IU (international units) four times a day is the recommended dose for children – are often inadequate to reduce this growth; for an infant, 500,000 IU four times a day will do the trick.
- A nystatin cream (prescribed by your doctor) can also be applied directly to the rash. Aloe vera gel is an effective alternative.

Thrush

This is a painful mouth infection caused by an overgrowth of yeast. The symptoms – white patches adhering to the mucous lining of the mouth, tongue or throat – may look like tonsillitis. Your doctor can make an accurate diagnosis from a throat or white-patch culture.

Nystatin, the anti-yeast drug, is routinely prescribed for thrush. I recommend following the same general course of treatment I outlined above for nappy rash.

Your baby may have caught thrush from your nipples, if you are breast-feeding; this is a common site for yeast infections. Ask your doctor to check if this is so; you don't want to reinfect your baby. Treatment is similar to that outlined above.

RECURRENT INFECTIONS

Recurrent ear infections

These are usually caused by allergy-inflamed tissue. Swollen tissue prevents fluid from draining out of the middle ear, and this dammed-up fluid becomes a breeding ground for bacteria. I usually see children with this problem when they are four-to-eight years old, after they've had multiple infections and their doctors have recommended using tubes (grommets) to balance the air pressure on both sides of the eardrum, and possibly even operations to remove adenoids and/or tonsils. In my experience, the real problem is that these children are allergy prone and not receiving the EFAs – especially omega-3 – they need to keep their immune system in good shape. In addition, the antibiotics administered to combat the infection have killed off their normal intestinal bacteria, making room for an overgrowth of yeast. Often a child becomes allergic to *Candida*, leading to respiratory congestion that is usually misdiagnosed as a cold. Treatment varies with age. For infants under one year, I recommend the following:

• Avoid antibiotics unless a bacterial infection is definitely found. Bacterial infections – sore throat due to infection by streptococci bacteria ('strep throat'), bronchitis, pneumonia and middle-ear infection – usually cause fever, pain and/or shortness of breath. Antibiotics are effective against bacteria, but most colds, sore throats and coughs are caused by viruses, which do not respond to antibiotics.

• If your child does have a bacterial infection and takes antibiotics, ask your doctor to prescribe him 500,000 IU of nystatin suspension four times a day, continuing for a week after he's off the antibiotic. This will do nothing but kill yeast. If your child has had antibiotics and now has allergy problems, I recommend one additional month of nystatin treatment.

• Give him *Lactobacillus bifidus* to restore his normal intestinal bacteria.

• Temporarily delete all sugar from his diet, including fruits and fruit juices. If he is on a cow's milk formula, switch to soya. Eliminate all other cow's-milk-based foods such as yoghurt. Once his congestion clears up, you can reintroduce these foods to see which ones he can tolerate.

● Give him 1 to 2 teaspoons (5–10 ml) of linseed oil a day or 2 to 4 teaspoons (10–20 ml) of walnut oil.

● Give him 500 to 1000 mg of vitamin C a day. In high doses, vitamin C is anti-allergenic. If he gets diarrhoea, cut back his dosage.

● Make sure his diet is rich in zinc, iron and vitamin A. We get most of our vitamin A in the form of carotene (the orange pigment in carrots and in many green, red and yellow vegetables). Carotene is an excellent anti-oxidant, but to stimulate the immune system, it has to be converted to retinol, or true vitamin A. I have found that many children with recurrent infections seem to have problems making this conversion and they need to eat foods that contain retinol. Good sources are egg yolks and liver, combined with vitamin C to enhance iron absorption. Feed them daily for a month, then cut back to twice a week so you don't overdose your baby with vitamin A.

Cod-liver oil is a good source of both vitamin A and omega-3s, but to avoid a vitamin A overdose, don't give it to your baby if he is also eating liver.

Alexi was a child whose problems started with ear infections. He had been formula-fed, and did well until, at six months, he had one or two ear infections and was given antibiotics. After these treatments, he began spitting up hard globs of mucus three or four times a day. When I saw him, at eleven months, he was irritable and cranky. He was eating jars of baby foods and had become very constipated. I switched him from a milk to a soya formula, and his condition improved. When his mother cut out commercial baby food and puréed his vegetables herself, his spitting up decreased by 90 per cent. When he was put back on commercial foods, it returned.

I decided that the antibiotics that he had been given might have started his problem by killing the 'good' bacteria in his intestine and allowing a yeast overgrowth. That, in turn, had probably contributed to a food allergy. I recommended a *Lactobacillus bifidus* supplement and a short course of nystatin to kill the yeast. Alexi's whole problem cleared up.

Excess mucus, coughing, congestion

First, make sure there are no smokers in the house. Then, if you've done a food trial, give your baby the EFAs – especially omega-3 – that he probably lacks. One to 2 teaspoons (5–10 ml) a day of linseed oil or 1 tablespoon (15 ml) of walnut oil or cod-liver oil should do it.

In addition, follow the recommendations for supplements detailed above under 'Recurrent ear infections'. Excess mucus, coughing and congestion can easily turn into a respiratory or ear infection.

Recurrent respiratory infections

These may also originate in allergic symptoms and can be treated in the same way as recurrent ear infections.

Nothing can compare with the first year of your child's life, but now he is about to become a toddler. Nothing will compare with this, either: he's about to start showing you that he's an individual with a mind of his own. The next two chapters will deal with this remarkable period.

Ages 1 to 5:
The Supernourished Toddler
and Young Child

5

Toddlers can be awkward. This is the age when the word *no* enters their vocabulary, and they love to use it. It's perfectly natural. Toddlers are beginning to assert their individuality, their sense of being a separate self, and saying *no* is their way of setting boundaries.

As a smart parent, you will learn how to outflank, rather than confront, your toddler or young child over getting dressed, going to bed and all the daily occasions in between. Good strategies are especially important when it comes to food, because if an all-out nutrition war is hard on you, it can be disastrous for your child's eating habits later in life.

There is one basic principle to remember when your toddler says *no* to food: *You control* what *she eats, and she controls* how much *she eats*. In practice, this means that it is not productive to tell a toddler, say, that she won't get a biscuit unless she eats everything on her plate. It may be tempting to say this when she refuses to eat her carrots, but if you give way to the temptation, the end result will be that she will think biscuits are one of the most important things in life, while eating carrots is pure punishment.

A good way to look at this problem is that a sweet is on the menu, and so are vegetables, or soup, or whatever. You decide the menu, and serve your toddler everything on it. She doesn't get to ask for something that's not on the menu. But if she really can't stand carrots that night, she can decide not to eat them. She will still get the sweet, because it's on the menu. And the chances are that, if eating carrots has not been made into a sore point, the next time you serve them, she will eat them with gusto. (It's a good idea to serve your toddler at the dinner table with the rest of the family, so she can learn that meals are sociable occasions, and that lots of people actually *like* carrots.)

Another way to deal with this problem – which partly results from the fact that children, like all of us, naturally like sweets – is to make sweets as nutritious as possible, so that when your toddler eats them, she is not just consuming sugars and non-essential fats, both of which can weaken her immune system. You will find plenty of home-tested, nutritious recipes in Chapter 10.

Your toddler's immune system is growing up along with her, and this means she will get infections – colds, sore throats, flu, earache. This sounds contradictory, because I have been promising that the nutritional guidelines you are following will bolster your child's defences. And they will. But you may recall that, in Chapter 1, I pointed out that a child's immune system has to be educated. The lymphocytes, those crucial white blood cells that send your child's other defensive cells into action, have to learn to recognize the thousands of germs, viruses, fungi and other microbes that invade everyone's body in the course of a lifetime.

Each infection your child gets now will serve to teach and strengthen her immune system, so that the next time that microbe invades, she won't get sick. The healthier her lymphocytes are, the faster they will learn – and the more quickly they will call out the cells that destroy invaders. With good nutrition and a well-regulated immune system, most of your child's infections should be relatively mild. So one of your jobs is to keep her white blood cells healthy by providing foods rich in EFAs and the key co-factor nutrients that help her body metabolize them. The end result of EFA metabolism is the prostaglandins that keep your child's defence system humming. You will also want to give your child a good supply of foods containing the anti-oxidants that fight the damage done to EFAs by free radicals, the 'sparks' given off when her body burns pollutants. And, of course, as much as possible, you will want to keep anti-nutrients such as sugar, partially hydrogenated fats, sodium and added phosphates out of your child's diet altogether. Anti-nutrients keep her body from metabolizing EFAs, so they are destructive to her immune system. (If you want to refresh your memory on all this, just reread Chapter 1.)

These preschool years are the last time you will have almost complete control over your child's diet. Once she starts going to school, and peer pressure becomes important to her, the temptations of junk foods will become very strong. But at this age, she is developing her tastes, and by feeding her nutritious foods that are naturally sweet, for example, you will help her develop a taste for them, rather than the sugar-loaded sweets and pastries she will inevitably encounter later on. (Contrary to popular mythology, well-nourished toddlers do not crave sweets, and will normally not stuff themselves with them. A psychologically conditioned craving for sweets is often developed later.) A palate accustomed to low-salt cooking will find most manufactured foods too salty, and a child who has grown up eating grilled, baked or stir-fried meat, poultry and fish may find fastfood hamburgers, chicken nuggets and deep-fried fish too greasy.

The biggest nutritional challenge facing you now is how to make sure your child gets enough of the important co-factor minerals and vitamins and the anti-oxidants, as well as certain other key nutrients. Your biggest concerns will be calcium, magnesium, iron, zinc and vitamin A – far too many toddlers are deficient in one or several of these. The solution is not as simple as, say, having your child drink a lot of milk to get calcium. As we shall see, this habit, which children have been traditionally encouraged to develop, does not, in fact, make good nutritional sense. But first, as always, we need to look at those crucial EFAs.

MAINTAINING THE EFAs

Your first concern in helping to bolster your child's immune system will be to maintain her supply of EFAs, especially the omega-3s in which children are commonly deficient. If you haven't already, you should add linseed oil to her diet at this point, in the following doses, depending on her age:

> One to two years: 1 teaspoon (5 ml) a day
> Two to three years: 2 teaspoons (10 ml) a day
> Three and up: 1 tablespoon (15 ml) a day

If food-grade linseed oil is unavailable, use twice the dosage of walnut oil or half the dosage of cod-liver oil.

If your child's skin and hair have become dry and dull, these amounts of linseed oil should do the trick. If both hair and skin don't soon regain their natural lustre, you can double the doses. Many toddlers and young children can swallow a tablespoon (15 ml) of linseed oil like medicine, if it is followed immediately by food or juice. You can mix linseed oil into juice (stir well and have her drink it quickly, before the oil and juice separate). Or you can use linseed or walnut oil in dressings, spreads and for baking. (*See* pp. 13–14 for ideas, and Chapter 10 for recipes.)

If your child's skin and hair don't improve after this trial, the chances are she needs omega-6 EFAs. Stop the oil you are using and give her an equivalent dose of cold-pressed safflower oil instead. (Safflower oil, too, can be used in dressings, spreads and for baking.)

BEYOND LINSEED OIL

At this age, you can begin to introduce your child to other sources of omega-3 EFAs. Walnut butter is sometimes hard to find, but it makes a fine substitute for peanut butter. The oil in peanuts is unsaturated, but because of the way the fatty acids are arranged, it promotes cholesterol accumulation – one reason I don't recommend peanut oil for cooking. And commercial brands of peanut butter are often partially hydrogenated. Partial hydrogenation, you will recall, makes perfectly good oils poison to your child's immune system by interfering with the metabolism of EFAs. Walnuts can be ground and used as a garnish, as can linseed.

Now is the time, too, to introduce your child to fish, which is very rich in EFAs. Serve cooked, soft, moist fish twice a week. Start with such bland fish as cod and haddock – you can slowly encourage your youngster to try the stronger, more oily, EFA-rich fish such as tuna and salmon. Avoid fresh-water fish and shoreline bottom-feeders such as flounder and sole because of possible PCB accumulation.

If you are worried about mercury contamination of fish, let me reassure you. Studies show that mercury levels in salmon have stayed constant over the years. Whatever amounts of mercury are found in these deep-water ocean fish occur naturally.

Fresh tuna is far superior to canned, which has had some of its EFAs removed or destroyed in processing. Look for fish that is dark rose in colour and has a moist surface. If it looks and feels dry, or is bleached white, or its flesh is separating into segments, the tuna is no longer fresh – pass it by.

Don't forget another excellent source of EFAs: beans, especially soya, kidney and haricot. Beans and tofu (soyabean curd) are quadruply valuable, because they supply protein, minerals and calcium, too. If you are just becoming acquainted with the wonderfully versatile tofu, you should know that there are two kinds: hard and soft. Hard tofu, sold in bricks, has the consistency of a moderately firm cheese. You can cut it into chunks and broil or stir-fry it, or simmer it in a soup or stew. Soft tofu has the consistency of a creamy yoghurt and can be used in all the same ways as yoghurt, in spreads, toppings and shakes, or mixed with fruit. Since tofu is tasteless, it will accept almost any flavour and can be used with any kind of sauce. (*See* recipes in Chapter 10.) Tofu is available from healthfood shops and from an increasing number of supermarkets.

DECREASING ANTI-OXIDANTS

No one who eats food can avoid eating pollutants. Chemical toxins in foods are a major public-health problem today. No food is immune: grains, nuts, seeds, fruit and vegetables, unless organically grown, are treated with pesticides. 'Factory-raised' chickens, like non-organically raised cattle, are treated with antibiotics (and, in some countries, notably the United States, with hormones) and eat feed treated with pesticides and preservatives. Most seafood contains mercury. Even mother's milk contains PCBs.

Your child's anti-oxidant defence system works to protect her body from damage caused by such environmental pollutants in foods. It also protects her white blood cells from damage in the performance of their duties, and prevents damage to EFAs from the free radicals generated when her cells burn off pollutants.

To do its job, the anti-oxidant defence system needs particular vitamins (A, C, E, B_2 [riboflavin], B_3 [nicotinic acid]) and minerals (zinc, copper, manganese, sulphur, selenium). Your child will need a diet rich in anti-oxidants all her life; now is a good time to start her on them.

The best food sources of anti-oxidants are:

- *Vitamin A:* carrots, sweet potatoes, red peppers, pumpkin, broccoli, liver
- *Vitamin C:* citrus fruits, tomatoes, strawberries, red peppers, broccoli
- *Vitamin E:* oatmeal, sunflower seeds, hazelnuts, almonds, unrefined EFA-rich oils
- *Vitamin B_2:* dairy products
- *Vitamin B_3:* whole grains (except maize)
- *Zinc:* liver, meat, oysters
- *Copper:* fish, sesame seeds, tofu, kidney beans
- *Manganese:* brown rice, oatmeal, split peas, almonds, peanuts, hazelnuts, walnuts, blackberries
- *Selenium:* fish, shellfish, oatmeal
- *Sulphur:* fish and other protein-rich foods, including meat and eggs

Liver

Some parents have expressed concern about liver in the diet because they've heard that this organ concentrates the toxins, hormones and antibiotics to which an animal is exposed in its lifetime. It is true that the liver, an organ whose function is to remove toxic substances from the body, will contain pollutants. But liver is an important source of zinc, vitamin A and other anti-oxidants as well as iron, and in my experience, its nutritional value far outweighs the dangers of any toxins it contains.

The best source of liver is cattle raised under 'organic' conditions – pasture grazed, with no feed laced with hormones or antibiotics. No super-markets as yet supply this type of meat, but the Real Meat Company (whose animals are fed on feed containing no growth promoters or antibiotics) sells its products in over 40 outlets in the South and South-west. Other firms selling organic meat are Natural Farms and the Pure Meat Company.

THE MIGHTY MINERALS

THE CALCIUM CONNECTION

Your child is going to need lots of calcium in these years as her bones grow and she uses her legs more and more to walk, run and climb. She will need about 600 to 800 mg a day.

Dairy products are the best sources of calcium, but believe it or not, *it is possible to drink too much milk or eat too much yoghurt.* Milk and yoghurt are very poor in iron and zinc, and in large quantities, they will replace in your child's diet foods that supply those essential nutrients. What's more, calcium blocks zinc and iron absorption. The result of too much milk or too many milk products in the diet is usually iron or zinc deficiency. A total of 16 fluid ounces (460 ml) of dairy products – milk, yoghurt, and/or cottage cheese – each day is plenty. Although yoghurt is preferred because some varieties contain *Lactobacillus acidophilus*, I wouldn't insist that a child eat yoghurt instead of drinking milk if she prefers the latter.

Enough milk or yoghurt is important, and I feel that unless your child has a specific intolerance or is allergic to milk, she should have milk products. It is hard to get enough calcium into her if you remove the best sources. Besides, milk provides protein and vitamin A, an important co-factor nutrient in metabolizing EFAs. Whole milk is a source of omega-6 EFAs.

Good non-dairy sources of calcium are beans (don't forget tofu) and almonds. Your child might enjoy bean soup, split-pea soup, chilli with kidney beans, bean salads and tortillas, which are made with calcium-rich lime (and are now available ready-made from some supermarkets). Chickpeas make a good snack.

Dark-green leafy vegetables such as spinach, broccoli, kale and parsley contain calcium, too, but they also contain oxalic acid, which may interfere with calcium absorption. I don't recommend dark-green vegetables as a source of calcium at this age. Broccoli and kale provide vitamins A and C, though, and are worth eating for that reason. If your child has a problem with the relatively bitter taste of dark-green leafy vegetables, try steaming broccoli florets *very* briefly (1 to 2 minutes) and serving them with a tahini or tofu dip. This will both enhance their flavour and make them a finger food, much more fun to eat.

Because some nutritionists advise against the use of cow's milk, I have composed the following list. It will show you how hard it is to give a child

600 mg of calcium a day without including 16 fluid ounces (460 ml) of milk or yoghurt in the diet:

CALCIUM SOURCES

FOOD	QUANTITY	CALCIUM (mg)
Spinach, cooked	3½ oz (100 g)	600
Milk	8 fl. oz (230 ml)	288
Yoghurt	8 fl. oz (230 ml)	174
Tofu	4 fl. oz (115 ml)	128
Chickpeas, cooked	7 oz (200 g)	128
Cottage cheese	4 oz (112 g)	67
Parmesan cheese	1 tbsp (5 g)	61
Almond butter	1 oz (30 g)	43
Tortilla	1	42
Bean soup (homemade)	4 fl. oz (115 ml)	41
Spring greens, cooked	1½ oz (40 g)	34
Broccoli, raw	1½ oz (45 g)	34
Cabbage, cooked	3 oz (90 g)	34

Should your child take a calcium supplement

If she doesn't consume 16 fluid ounces (460 ml) of dairy foods or their equivalent every day, your child will do well to take one. She'll tolerate calcium carbonate supplements nicely in liquid or chewable form. Although I don't recommend this form for adult women, children usually have enough stomach acid to absorb it if it's given with food.

Calcium carbonate is usually derived from ground oyster shells – check the label, and avoid calcium from bone meal or dolomite, which may be contaminated with lead and other toxic metals.[1]

Don't overdo the amount you give your child – too much may interfere with her body's ability to absorb magnesium, iron and zinc. If she consumes no milk, yoghurt or cheese, 600 mg a day of supplemental calcium is plenty, unless she has one of the rare diseases that interferes with calcium metabolism. Give her the supplements with meals to enhance their absorption.

MAGNESIUM

At this stage, your growing child needs about 5 mg of magnesium per pound of body weight, or about 100 to 250 mg a day. Magnesium is an important co-factor mineral in the metabolism of EFAs, and a deficiency can contribute to the severity of allergies. So you will want to help your child develop a taste for magnesium-rich foods: nuts, seeds, grains such as oats and buckwheat (although buckwheat, technically, is not a true grain), pulses (cooked and in salads), tofu, fish and nut butters (unsalted, with no sugar added). Skip peanut butter or limit it to once a week – it can raise cholesterol levels and interfere with your child's EFA metabolism. Give her almond or walnut butter instead.

Tofu is an excellent meat substitute as well as providing magnesium and calcium.

IRON AND ZINC: TWO FOR THE BLOOD CELLS

Iron

This is a critical nutrient for toddlers and other young children, who need it for the production of the white blood cells that make up their immune system's army, as well as for the red blood cells that carry oxygen in their blood. Ironically, children who drink lots of milk can easily become iron-deficient, because milk contains very little iron and because calcium can block their body's ability to absorb iron from other foods.

Shellfish such as oysters are excellent sources of iron and zinc, but they are shoreline feeders and so, unlike deep-water ocean fish, may contain pollutants. *Never serve them raw.* Chop them up and cook them in a stew.

The best animal source of iron is liver (*see* p. 81 for more information). Any danger to the toddler from too much vitamin A can be eliminated by limiting liver to no more than 4 ounces (115 g) a week, unless under a doctor's direction.

Sesame butter (tahini) contains significant amounts of iron, but the body doesn't digest iron from vegetable sources very well. Vitamin C enhances absorption, so serve tahini in a dip or sauce with broccoli or sweet red peppers. Sunflower seeds, another useful source of iron, could accompany oranges, grapefruit, strawberries or tomatoes.

Raisins are a good source of iron, but they are also a good source of tooth decay because they stick to the teeth. Children should brush their teeth after eating any dried fruit.

As you will see from the list that follows, it's not easy for children to meet their need for iron, so iron-poor junk foods have no place in these diets – food must supply much more than just calories.

IRON SOURCES

FOOD	QUANTITY	IRON (mg)
Meats, cooked	2 oz (55 g)	
Liver		6
Beef		2
Pork		2
Lamb		2
Poultry		1
Oysters, cooked	2 oz (55 g)	10
Fish, cooked	2 oz (55 g)	1
Sesame butter	1 tbsp (15 ml)	1
Egg yolk	1	1
Black treacle	1 tbsp (15 ml)	3
Raisins	½ oz (15 g)	9

Zinc

This mineral promotes the growth and development of your child's white blood cells, especially the lymphocytes, those T- and B-cells that identify invading germs and send out antibodies to zap the invaders. Zinc also helps keep the thymus gland healthy and productive. This gland is where T [for thymus]-cells are produced and receive their basic training. What's more, zinc plays key roles in overall growth and in the development of the brain. Unfortunately, many children don't get enough of this vital mineral.

The all-time best source of zinc is Atlantic oysters – your child needs about 10 mg a day, and 1 ounce (30 g) of Atlantic oysters will give him over 20 mg. No other source comes close. However, beef, nuts and seeds such as sesame and pumpkin contain some zinc.

The following are the best food sources of zinc:

ZINC SOURCES

FOOD	AMOUNT	ZINC (mg)
Animal		
Crabmeat, steamed	1 oz (30 g)	1.2
Beef liver	1 oz (30 g)	1.0
Egg	1	1.0
Beef, minced	1 oz (30 g)	0.9
Turkey (dark)	1 oz (30 g)	0.9

FOOD	AMOUNT	ZINC (mg)
Animal		
Chicken (dark)	1 oz (30 g)	0.5
Turkey (light)	1 oz (30 g)	0.4
Chicken (light)	1 oz (30 g)	0.2
Fish, moist	1 oz (30 g)	0.2
Vegetable		
Pumpkin seeds	2 oz (55 g)	2.0
Kidney beans, cooked	5½ oz (160 g)	1.6
Almonds	1 oz (30 g)	1.0
Black treacle	1 tbsp (15 ml)	0.9
Peanuts	1 oz (25 g)	0.75
Walnuts	⅔ oz (20 g)	0.6

To get 10 mg of zinc a day, a toddler might eat these foods:

FOOD	ZINC (mg)
3 oz (85 g) turkey	3.6
2 tbsp (30 ml) almond butter	1.0
2¾ oz (80 g) kidney beans	0.8
1¼ oz (35 g) oatmeal (porridge), cooked	0.6
2 slices wholewheat bread	1.2
4½ oz (130 g) brown rice	1.8
2¾ oz (80 g) peas	0.6
4½ oz (130 g) carrots	0.3
1½ oz (45 g) broccoli	0.1
Total	10.0

Your toddler can get half of what she needs from such unrefined, low-zinc foods as fish, brown rice, vegetables and beans; the other half should come from such high-zinc foods as poultry, nuts, seeds, eggs and meat.

Although wheat bran contains zinc, the phytate in the bran blocks its absorption, which is why I don't advocate it for toddlers. *I also don't advocate zinc supplementation*, except under medical supervision. At any age, too much zinc will block iron and selenium uptake and lower body levels of copper and manganese, two other vital minerals.

Studies of children with recurrent infections show that they have lower blood levels of iron and zinc than do healthy children. These low levels persist even between the children's bouts with infection, suggesting that zinc and iron deficiencies may cause susceptibility to infection.[2] This is what happened to Joshua.

Joshua was three years old when I saw him. He seemed to catch everything that was going around – colds, diarrhoea, bronchitis. If someone in the neighbourhood had an infection, Josh caught it. He'd be sick for a week or two, then recover. Fortunately, his doctor was not very keen on antibiotics, which can do harm to young children. (And could not have done any good against his infections anyway since they were all virus-based.)

When I examined Josh, he was between infections and seemed to be a healthy, active youngster with no evidence of allergies. He didn't eat a lot of sugar, and his parents, who knew something about nutrition, served him few red meats. Josh liked milk, and got about half his calories from whole milk, yoghurt and cottage cheese. He certainly didn't seem to be allergic to milk, but his diet was clearly low in zinc and iron. Sure enough, I found white spots on his fingernails, a sign of zinc – and sometimes of iron – deficiency. Josh wasn't anaemic, but a blood test showed that he had a low level of ferritin, the protein that stores iron in the body.

To confirm a zinc deficiency, we analysed a sample of Josh's hair. (Hair mineral analysis has become controversial because of abuse by irresponsible practitioners, but it is a proven method for assessing zinc status. It is also far less traumatic to a toddler to snip a few hairs from his head than it is to draw blood.) Josh's hair zinc was quite low.

Liver and red meat are good sources of both iron and zinc, but Josh's parents did not want to serve more of them. To encourage him to eat a wider variety of foods, I advised his parents to limit his total consumption of milk, yoghurt and cottage cheese to 16 fluid ounces (460 ml) a day. Then I put him on liquid iron and zinc supplements. He took these for four months, at meal times, until the spots disappeared from his nails.

At that point, we re-analysed Josh's diet. His parents had been adding pumpkin seeds to his cereal and giving him more fish and poultry. Together with less milk, this regimen had significantly raised the amounts of zinc and iron in his diet, and I took him off the supplements.

After two more months, Josh's immune system had grown much stronger and more active. His infections became milder, shorter and, finally, fewer. He even escaped a few flu epidemics that swept his neighbourhood.

Why not continue the zinc and iron supplements indefinitely? Because while children need the right amount of iron and zinc, too much can be harmful. Population studies show that high iron and zinc levels are associated with increased risk of cancer in adulthood. Experimental studies with animals suggest a method by which this could work: too much zinc may induce cancer by depleting the body's level of manganese and selenium. Excess iron also lowers manganese levels.

Good nutrition derives from a balance, not megadoses, of nutrients.

VITAMIN A

Vitamin A serves both as a co-factor nutrient, helping the enzymes in your child's body metabolize EFAs, and as an anti-oxidant, protecting his white blood cells and other cells from attacks by free radicals and from overheating while killing germs or burning off toxins. It is also crucial to healthy skin and good vision.

A recent study at the US National Institutes of Health discovered that a single virus infection (in this case, chicken pox) depletes the vitamin A levels of healthy children for several months.[3] The RDAs in the US and UK* for vitamin A are:

	AGES	DOSAGE (international units/day)
US RDA	1–3	2000
	4–5	2500
UK RDA	1–6	1000

The best sources of vitamin A are orange, red, yellow and deep-green vegetables such as carrots, sweet potatoes, spinach and broccoli, and red, orange and yellow fruits such as melon and apricots. These all contain carotene, an orange pigment that your child's body metabolizes into retinol, the active form of vitamin A. Since her body controls the rate at which carotene is converted, and does not make more retinol than she needs, vitamin A from vegetable sources is never toxic.

Animal sources of vitamin A – such as liver, whole milk and egg yolks – contain retinol, so it is possible for your child to get too much vitamin A from these sources. Even so, while toddlers are more susceptible to vitamin A toxicity than older children, amounts of retinol under 10,000 units a day are not likely to be toxic, even for them.

As the following lists show, it is not hard to give your child foods that contain enough vitamin A for her needs – you just have to know which ones to serve.

---

* The UK Department of Health now prefers measurements of vitamins A and D to be expressed in micrograms (μg). To calculate this, multiply the number of international units (IUs) by 0.3.

RETINOL SOURCES

FOOD	AMOUNT	RETINOL (international units)
Egg yolk	1	600
Liver		
beef or calf	1 oz (30 g)	10,000
chicken	1 oz (30 g)	3,500
Whole milk	8 fl. oz (230 ml)	350
Cod-liver oil	1 tbsp (15 ml)	10,000

CAROTENE SOURCES

FOOD	AMOUNT	CAROTENE (international units)
Vegetables		
Carrots, cooked	4½ oz (130 g)	8,700
Sweet potato	1 small	8,100
Carrot, raw	4¼ oz (120 g)	8,000
Spinach, cooked	3½ oz (100 g)	3,400
Tomato juice	4 fl. oz (115 ml)	800
Broccoli, cooked	1½ oz (45 g)	600
Tomato	1 medium	250
Fruits		
Mango	1	11,000
Watermelon	8 oz (225 g) wedge	5,000
Cantaloupe	4 oz (115 g) wedge	3,400
Apricots (fresh)	9 oz (260 g)	2,200

SEVEN COMMON QUESTIONS ABOUT FEEDING YOUNG CHILDREN

The pages that follow will provide some simple, commonsense answers to the questions I am most frequently asked about the general care and feeding of toddlers and young children.

DO THEY NEED FIBRE?

If you are following my nutritional guidelines, you don't need to worry about whether your child is getting enough fibre. Young children have small stomachs, and high-fibre foods are bulky. If your child eats oats, some beans and other pulses and some nut butters, plus a variety of vegetables, he will get all the fibre he needs. Wait until he is older before thinking about giving him such concentrated fibre foods as bran.

WHAT ABOUT VEGETARIAN DIETS?

Some people think that a vegetarian diet is good because it avoids the fat and toxins in meats. But there are many reports of single and multiple nutritional deficiencies among vegetarian children, most commonly vitamin B_{12}, zinc, iron and protein. Although many authorities on vegetarian diets focus on combining grains, seeds, nuts, beans and dairy products in high-protein dishes, most do not adequately cover other nutrients. (The worst-nourished patients I've seen are casual vegetarians: they avoid animal foods but don't make the effort to include mineral- and protein-rich plant foods.)

Macrobiotic diets are low in toxins because they include a very limited range of foods, but they are also low in nutrients, and can be severely damaging to children unless they include fish and soya products as sources of protein, zinc, iron and vitamin B_{12}.

WHAT ARE THE BEST SNACKS FOR YOUNG CHILDREN?

All children like snacks, and in addition to three nutritionally balanced meals each day, an active child will need two or three nutritionally sound snacks. A good way to think about snacks is that they provide a handy way to give your child the nutrients he doesn't get in his regular meals – you can even think of them as 'mini-meals' that provide a mix of protein, carbohydrates and fat.

Many parents think a piece of fruit is a perfect snack. It's not. Why? Because an apple or pear won't be enough to keep your child satisfied until the next meal. Milk and yoghurt provide the right nutrients and are filling enough to keep the most active child happy until mealtime. Their big plus, of course, is calcium. In fact, snacks are the perfect way to fill a toddler's daily calcium needs. Even though it's liquid, milk is really more a food than a drink, and a child who drinks it with meals may find he has little room left for other foods. But as the perfect snack, milk offers protein, EFAs and vitamin A as well as calcium. Give milk at snack time, not at meals.

With a glass of milk, you can serve low-sugar oatmeal-sesame biscuits, a homemade sugar-free muesli bar or a dried fruit-and-nut bar (*see* recipes in chapter 10). Or try carrot sticks dipped in almond butter, or a wholewheat pita bread pizza. As an alternative to milk, mix plain yoghurt with fresh or frozen berries and chopped nuts, and serve tofu in a strawberry smoothie (*see* recipe).

ARE CONVENIENCE FOODS OK?

As we saw in Chapter 1, most manufactured foods are loaded with fats, sugar and/or salt, all anti-nutrients and all destructive to your child's immune system. But these days, it's virtually impossible to avoid using some convenience foods, such as cereal and canned foods.

● *Cereals.* Commercial cold cereals, including bran and muesli ingredients, are usually loaded with sugar and salt, and are often made with partially hydrogenated vegetable oils as well. These are particularly lethal because they contain artificial unsaturated fatty acids that block EFA metabolism. Luckily, it's easy to make a big batch of your own low-sugar muesli; my recipe is in Chapter 10.

If you're really pressed for time, some commercial cereals are low in sugar: plain Cheerios (available at Safeways supermarkets), Shredded Wheat (which contains neither sugar nor added salt), puffed wheat, puffed rice, Alpen, Special K. You don't have to worry about the fibre in these cereals; your healthy toddler can handle it well. Unfortunately, most of these cereals are loaded with salt, containing 150 to 300 mg of sodium per ounce (30 g). Two ounces (55 g) a day is not a problem, but if your child eats more cereal, these may significantly raise sodium intake.

● *Canned foods.* The problem with these is that, in addition to being full of salt and/or sugar, the seams of the tins are soldered with lead, which can leach into the food. It's much better to use foods packed in glass. In any case, *never* store opened canned food in the tin. Transfer it to a glass jar or plastic container and refrigerate. And limit the use of tinned items to once a week. Canned meats and fish can be used occasionally, and some vegetables and fruits are now being canned without added salt and/or sugar.

● *Convenience health foods.* Watch out for these. As we saw above, commercial mueslis are full of partially hydrogenated vegetable oil and often contain sugar and salt. Muesli bars are too. Products labelled 'low-calorie' usually contain as many calories *and* as many additives as other manufactured foods – they're just more expensive. In healthfood shops, though, you can usually find whole-grain breads and biscuits made without preservatives or partially hydrogenated vegetable oils. The Scandinavian crisp breads sold in supermarkets generally contain no added fats or preservatives; check the labels. Wholewheat pita is also good.

● *Do-it-yourself convenience foods.* The best convenience foods are the ones you make yourself, because you'll know exactly what goes into them. You can keep fastfoods on hand by 'batch-cooking' – cooking up a big batch of food and then storing it in portion-size quantities in the freezer, if you have one.

SHOULD YOU TAKE A YOUNG CHILD TO McDONALD'S?

Tempting as they are when you're pressed for time, avoid both fastfood places and pizza parlours. Most fastfood places fry or deep-fry their food with partially hydrogenated vegetable oil, a double threat because frying creates the free radicals that damage your child's immune system and other cells. Pizza is all right if you can get the real thing, made with real cheese and fresh tomatoes. But today most pizza is made with imitation cheese and tomato sauce. Imitation cheese is concocted with partially hydrogenated vegetable oil flavoured to taste like cheese; imitation tomato sauce is an artificially coloured, tomato-flavoured chemical soup.

The one exception to this ban on fastfood restaurants is Spud-U-Like, where all the dishes available are based on the good, honest baked potato.

WHAT IF ALL THE PARENTS TAKE THEIR KIDS TO McDONALDS?

There is no question that eating is an important occasion for socializing and, for young children, an important experience in socialization. But for the most part, there is no reason to compromise your high standards of nutrition. You can pack a picnic basket and take it to the park or playground. Your child can meet other children her age and perhaps even ask them to share her snack.

If you visit another home with your youngster and inappropriate foods are served for a meal or snack, you can ask whether something more appropriate could be substituted. If you discuss your child-feeding philosophy with the other adults there, you may find that they agree with you! If you meet some defensiveness, it may come from confusion; with a few minutes' discussion, you can probably clarify the situation and hit upon one or more foods your hosts have on hand that will suit your child's needs. Good nutrition isn't difficult; it's simply a matter of making the right choices and declining what's not appropriate. In any case, you never need to defend your methods to another parent. In a pinch, you can simply state that you feed your child in a certain way because you believe it's healthy and nourishing.

Which brings us back to those all but inevitable visits to the local fastfood restaurant. In fact, since you're providing your child with good nutrition every day, it won't hurt her to compromise perhaps once a week by having a slice of pizza or a Big Mac with the other kids. Socialization, after all, is often a matter of compromise. The main thing is that she is eating properly as a matter of habit. Too many other children eat poorly as a matter of habit; for them, fastfood is just one more item in an already poor diet.

HOW DO YOU HANDLE A PICKY EATER, OR A CHILD WHO WILL ONLY EAT ONE THING?

Toddlers are particularly quirky about food as about many other things, and there's no point in making an issue out of it. Don't threaten or bribe yours or capitulate to requests for changes in the menu. Most of all, don't panic. There's no point in asking your two-year-old what she wants to eat. Just provide the healthy foods she needs, and let her eat as much of them as she wants. She won't starve; eventually, she'll eat.

You can help by serving foods that look good and taste good. Be creative. If she won't drink milk, add milk or yoghurt to soup, cereal, ice lollies or smoothies (see Chapter 10). If she won't eat vegetables, mash or cream them into soups or stews. if she will only eat soft or sweet foods, you can mash or purée 'sweet' vegetables: parsnips, carrots or peas. Or you can mix something sweet and nutritious, such as orange juice, into her food.

If she's partial to salty foods, try mixing something salty but nutritious, such as cheese, into her food. You can flavour foods with such herbs or spices as fresh parsley, cinnamon, nutmeg or ginger. Almost everything tastes better with a sprinkle of lemon juice.

If you decide to add salt to anything, use sea salt; it not only tastes better, it's better for your child because it's rich in magnesium. Magnesium-enriched salt is another choice.

If she only wants to drink milk, you have to limit her to 16 fluid ounces (460 ml) a day; sooner or later, she'll get hungry and eat other things.

A CHILD'S MEAL PLAN

Planning meals for toddlers and young children involves some of the same considerations you use in planning meals for adults or older children: you want to serve a variety of foods, including, whenever possible, something your child really likes. Serving different-coloured foods is an attractive way to get nutritional variety, as though nature had chosen colour with this in mind. For instance, try to serve one green and one yellow, orange or red vegetable at both lunch and supper. If you start your child on crisp, crunchy salads and vegetable snacks, she will develop a taste for fresh raw vegetables.

• Give your child small quantities of several different foods at each meal. That way, she can ask for more if she particularly likes one thing. She will also feel that she has more control over how much she eats.

• Plan desserts as an integral, nutritious part of the meal, not as a junk-food 'treat'.

• Limit your child's intake of added sugar to just 1 teaspoon (5 ml) a day. This includes sugar you or a manufacturer adds as an ingredient in other foods.

Cooking utensils and food storage

Don't cook with aluminium, especially acid foods such as tomato sauce. You can actually see spaghetti sauce etch the aluminium out of pans. I like cast iron the best for cookware. Well-seasoned cast iron is easy to maintain, cooks evenly and adds iron to food. Heatproof glass and porcelain are also non-toxic.

The only non-toxic food wrap is grease-proof paper. Many brands of clingfilm contain potentially carcinogenic plasticizers (although some supermarket chains now sell safe 'non-PVC' or 'plasticizer-free' clingfilm, Bejam and Waitrose among them), and aluminium foil can be toxic unless you line it with grease-proof paper. If you store food in plastic bags, wrap it in grease-proof paper first.

The following guidelines will provide your child with a healthful, nutritious diet that will help her develop strong resistance to infections, strong bones and a lifelong taste for foods that are both delicious and good for her.

FIVE MEALS A DAY

This is a good schedule for *active* toddlers and preschool children:

> Breakfast
> Mid-morning snack
> Lunch
> Mid-afternoon snack
> Dinner

FOODS TO INCLUDE

Food	Serving size	Frequency
Milk or yoghurt	16 fl oz (460 ml)	Daily, no more than this. (Limit hard cheese to three 2 oz/55g servings a week.)
Meat	2 oz/55 g (a serving size roughly 2 × 2 × ¼ in/5 × 5 × 0.6 cm)	Once a week
Poultry	2 oz (roughly 2 × 2 × ¼ in/5 × 5 × 0.6 cm)	Up to three meals a week
Fish	2 oz (roughly 2 × 2 × ¼ in/5 × 5 × 0.6 cm)	Two meals a week, minimum; more if possible
Egg	1	One a day
Nut butter	2 tbsp (30 ml)	Daily
Beans	5½ oz (160 g)	Two meals a week, at least
Tofu	3 oz (85 g)	Two meals a week, at least
Fruit (emphasize fruits high in vitamin C, such as oranges, grapefruit or berries in season)	4½ oz (130 g)	Three servings daily
Vegetables (emphasize those high in vitamins A and C, such as tomatoes and broccoli)	2 tbsp (30 ml)	Six servings daily
Whole-grain bread	½ slice	
Cooked cereal	½ oz (15 g)	Three servings daily
Dry cereal	⅓ oz (10 g)	

BREAKFAST

This should be a high-protein meal. Leftovers from dinner would be good, but most children don't want fish or beans first thing in the morning. Here are some good high-protein breakfasts for children.

● *Cereal.* Porridge, the all-time favourite, is still the best. Don't add salt. Flavour it with fresh fruit or raisins. Milk is optional; if your child doesn't get enough during the day, add it now. You can flavour porridge with cinnamon, sunflower seeds and raisins to supply magnesium, calcium, zinc, vitamin A and iron.

Alternatives to porridge? Try homemade Swiss muesli (*see* recipes in Chapter 10), served with plain yoghurt or whole milk and fruit. This supplies calcium, magnesium and vitamins A and C. You can also serve homemade muesli (*see* Chapter 10) or the commercial cereals listed on page 91.

● *Egg.* Serve one boiled for at least eight minutes (to be sure to kill any salmonella that may be present), with wholewheat toast and orange juice. This supplies zinc, iron and vitamins A and C. As a general rule, don't serve fried or scrambled eggs; frying oxidizes the cholesterol, producing toxic by-products that can damage blood vessels.

Since eggs supply protein, iron and zinc, serve one a day unless your family has a history of cholesterol problems. This means that a close relative – mother, father, grandparent, uncle or aunt – has had a heart attack before the age of 60. However, always be sure to cook eggs thoroughly: salmonella poisoning can be deadly to a young child.

● *Wheat–soy pancakes.* (*See* recipe in Chapter 10.) These can be cooked in batches in advance and frozen.

● *Sesame waffles.* Served with applesauce (*see* Chapter 10), these supply magnesium and zinc.

Some other breakfast foods:
● *Bread and biscuits.* Use only those listing 100 per cent wholewheat flour (or other whole grains) as the first ingredient.
● *Spreads.* Nut butters are best. For sweetness, use unsweetened apple and pear spread instead of heavily sugared jams.
● *Beverages.* Orange juice is best; I recommend grapefruit juice, too. Unless they are fortified, other juices are lower in vitamin C. Serve milk only for snacks, not at mealtimes.

LUNCHES AND SNACKS
(mid-morning, noon and mid-afternoon)

Snack foods and lunch foods are basically interchangeable – in fact, think of lunch as another snack, equal in size to your child's mid-morning and mid-afternoon snacks. If she has had a good breakfast, and if she's likely to eat dinner, make lunches and snacks light and easy.

● *Soups.* Homemade are best. Canned or dried instant soups usually contain far too much salt and other anti-nutrients.

● *Sandwiches.* Use whole-grain breads. Use nut butters and fruit spreads. Limit fatty spreads such as mayonnaise to 1 teaspoon (5 ml) a day. (It's best to avoid most commercial mayonnaise altogether. You can get 'natural' mayonnaise, made with soya oil, in healthfood shops. Best of all, make your own, with linseed or walnut oil, but make sure that the eggs you use have been pasteurized or are from an impeccable source. *See* Chapter 10.)

Leftover meat, poultry or fish makes an excellent sandwich filling. Stay away from luncheon meats such as pressed ham or sausage – they're too high in salt and fat.

● *Yoghurt.* Add fresh fruit, chopped nuts or seeds and linseed or walnut oil.

● *Finger foods.* Youngsters love them. Carrot sticks are good plain or dabbed with nut butter, as are courgette sticks and blanched broccoli or cauliflower florets. The last two are especially high in vitamin C, as are peas, three-bean salad, green pepper strips and tomato wedges.

Don't serve potato crisps, which are too salty and soaked in heat-damaged oils.

A checklist of other possibilities *(see recipes in Chapter 10 for asterisked items)*:

● Low-salt cottage cheese with fresh fruit
● Nut butter on carrot sticks, or hummus* on celery
● Homemade muesli bar*
●. Homemade bean soup*: cook batch in advance and freeze in 4 fl. oz (115 ml) servings
● Tofu crisps (sautéed tofu) with sea salt
● Smoothies*: soft tofu or yoghurt puréed with banana or other fresh fruit and nut butter
● Whole-grain biscuits or wholewheat pita with nut butter and apple and pear spread, or with cheese
● Tuna or chicken mixed with homemade linseed or walnut oil mayonnaise*, served on whole-grain bread
● Mini-pizza made with a wholewheat muffin*, cheese and tomato*
● Any breakfast makes a fine lunch or snack; so do leftovers from dinner.

DINNER

Make dinner a light meal, too – it ensures a good night's sleep for everyone. Since it's usually the only meal at which the whole family eats together, include your child and give her the same foods as everyone else. Dinner should usually include the following foods:

- *Starch.* Brown rice, baked potato (mash your child's with a little milk, yoghurt or soft tofu), sweetcorn, whole-grain bread or kasha (roasted buckwheat). Kasha is rich in minerals, especially magnesium.
- *Vegetables.* Two, perhaps one green and one orange or yellow, for vitamins A and C. The best way to prepare vegetables is to steam them as briefly as possible until they are just tender. If necessary, mash them for your child. A small amount of grated cheese adds flavour.
- *Protein.* Limit red meat to one serving a week. Despite advertising to the contrary from meat producers, there is too much saturated fat even in lean red meat. Liver is the best choice because it is rich in folic acid and vitamin A, zinc and iron, all key nutrients for building a strong immune system. (*See* recipes in Chapter 10 for liver dishes.)

Poultry is a good source of protein, and the dark meat is rich in zinc and iron as well. The main problem with poultry is its contamination by hormones, antibiotics and pesticides. The best birds are free range and raised without hormones, antibiotics or pesticide-treated grain. Most supermarkets now sell free-range poultry (and eggs) but there is still no guarantee that they have not been injected or fed with growth promoters or preventive medication.

Serve seafood – shellfish or fish – two or three times a week. Seafood is low in saturated fat and high in omega-3 EFAs and important minerals. Stews and soups are tasty ways to serve seafood and are easy to prepare (*see* Chapter 10).

Serve beans and other pulses at least twice a week. Besides providing protein, they're excellent sources of magnesium, soluble fibre, minerals and *lectins*, starchy compounds that stimulate the immune cells of the intestine. You can add shredded or grated cheese for tanginess.

Some of the tastiest ways to prepare high-protein foods also provide important nutrients:

Bouillabaisse made with oysters, clams, cod, carrots, peas, tomatoes, potatoes or rice (*see* recipes in Chapter 10). Rich in EFAs, zinc, iron (shellfish), selenium (fish), vitamin A (carrots and tomatoes), and vitamin C (tomatoes). An excellent immune booster.

Grilled fish almondine with brown rice, lemon, broccoli, tomatoes and almonds. Provides magnesium, selenium and vitamins A and C.

Brown rice and pinto beans with sweet red peppers (*see* Chapter 10). Rich in magnesium and vitamins A and C.

Pasta and haricot beans with tomato (*see* Chapter 10). Supplies magnesium, folic acid and vitamins A and C.

Roast Poultry. Dark-meat turkey is the best; it's richest in zinc and iron. In the same oven, bake a sweet potato (the type with the orange flesh, available from West Indian grocers and, increasingly, from supermarkets) to provide vitamins A and C. Steam cauliflower or asparagus spears.

Stir-fried vegetables, such as carrots, broccoli florets, water chestnuts and Chinese cabbage; add tofu or sliced meat or poultry and bean sprouts (mung or adzuki); serve over white or brown rice. Supplies vitamin A, magnesium and protein. (*Note:* Young toddlers may have trouble with the crunchy vegetables, but should have no problem with tofu, rice and bean sprouts.)

DESSERTS

These are traditional after dinner. They should be a nutritious part of the meal, not a special treat. Don't use sweets as a bribe to get your child to eat other foods; that will just make them seem more important than they really are.

The following desserts are delicious and wholesome.

- *Homemade ice lollies.* Although they are messy, youngsters enjoy them. You can make your own very easily: Buy metal moulds, pour in plain juice with puréed or mashed fruit mixed with yoghurt, and freeze. Do not add sugar.
- *Fruit salad.* Orange and grapefruit slices for vitamin C, plus other fruits in season. For crunchiness and magnesium, top with chopped nuts. For texture, calcium and protein, top with yoghurt or soft tofu.
- *Fresh fruit in season.* Baked apple with cinnamon, natural (unsweetened) applesauce with raisins, berries topped with plain yoghurt and chopped nuts, or peaches over cottage cheese with sesame seeds.
- *Low-sugar pastries* made with whole-grain flour and dried fruit: sugar-free oatmeal raisin biscuits, apple–coconut muffins, spice cake (*see* recipes in Chapter 10).
- *Sugar-free pies* with whole-wheat crusts and cooked fresh or fruit–tofu fillings, like pumpkin–tofu pie (*see* recipes in Chaper 10).
- *Yoghurt sundae.* Blend yoghurt with banana or berries, top with mixed nuts, cinnamon or nutmeg. Chill.
- *Fruit-juice snow cone or frozen fruit juice ice lollies.*
- *Smoothies* (*see* recipes in Chapter 10).
- *Low-sugar tofu pudding* (*see* recipes in Chapter 10).

These desserts supply nutrients to complement the day's meals. If your child hasn't eaten much yoghurt or drunk much milk that day, choose one of the yoghurt or tofu recipes. If she hasn't eaten citrus fruits or tomatoes, choose a fruit dessert and include a citrus fruit. If she hasn't had much magnesium, choose a tofu- or nut-based recipe.

If you follow this diet plan carefully, your child will eat and drink an ample supply of the nutrients that, at this age, are most important both for growth and for a healthy immune system.

Nutritional First Aid
to Fight Childhood Illnesses

6

Toddlers are beginning to get out into the world, and inevitably they will come down with illnesses of one kind or another. Their immune systems are still meeting new challenges. Fortunately, most common childhood illnesses – stomach aches, colds, some recurrent bacterial infections, allergies, even chronic behavioural problems – respond very well to nutritional therapy. In fact, in many cases these problems are actually symptoms of nutritional deficits.

If your child has rough, dry skin or hair, is constipated and/or frequently gets stomach aches, colds, sore throats or ear infections, he probably has a nutritional problem. If his eyes are puffy or there are dark circles under them, if he has a persistent drippy nose or night-time cough, if he's over four years old but still constantly wets his bed, or if he has frequent mood changes, he may well have a food allergy.

Western society relies heavily on prescription and over-the-counter drugs, and in some cases, particularly with middle-ear infections, drugs are needed to clear up a problem. But drugs, especially antibiotics, can also create their own problems, and those can be most effectively dealt with through nutrition. In other cases, such as colds, reaching for the aspirin or paracetamol is not usually the best course, particularly with a toddler. Nutrition will do a better job. Your child will come out of his illness with a healthier immune system that will probably be able to fight off the next invasion of virus or bacteria.

In the pages that follow, I shall give you step-by-step procedures to follow for the most common childhood illnesses. But first, it's useful to know how to recognize simple nutritional deficiency.

SIGNS OF A SIMPLE NUTRITIONAL DEFICIENCY

A deficiency in a specific nutrient can announce itself with a single symptom. The cure is simple; refer to Chapter 5 and supply your child with the right amount of that nutrient:

SYMPTOM	POSSIBLE DEFICIENCY
Dry or rough skin or hair	EFAs
White spots on nails	Zinc or iron
Constipation	Magnesium or fibre
Craving for sweets	A sign not of a single deficiency but of general undernutrition

Well-fed, well-nourished children do not crave sweets. Conditioned, or psychological, cravings for sugar come later. Toddlers will eat a small amount of ice cream or sweets, but they won't stuff themselves. The solution to this problem is to read Chapter 5 and apply the principles of nutrition detailed there to your own child.

Still, youngsters are not immune to social pressures, especially TV advertising. So there will be times when your well-fed child will badger you for sweets. Don't give in. At home, give him the food *you* want him to eat, but don't force him to eat it. If you're in the supermarket and he spots a sugar-coated cereal or sweets he's seen on TV, move to another area. If you're in the checkout queue, try to ignore him. Or divert him; change the subject. Point out how interesting the checkout procedure is.

Now, let's look at some common childhood illnesses.

STOMACH ACHES

This is the commonest health problem among toddlers. The pain can range from relatively mild to excruciating, but the cure is usually simple. Investigators at McMaster University in Ontario, Canada studied digestive complaints in 149 healthy two-year-olds. Constipation was a chronic problem in 16 per cent, diarrhoea in 8 per cent and abdominal pain in 5 per cent. Altogether, 27 per cent had some kind of chronic intestinal disturbance. However, by the age of 40 months, only 5 per cent had intestinal problems. The main difference between affected and unaffected youngsters was in fluid consumption. Toddlers with digestive complaints consumed almost twice as much fluid, usually fruit juice, as toddlers without digestive complaints. The investigators speculated that the high carbohydrate-to-fat ratio of fruit juices may not be tolerated by some toddlers below the age of three years. As discussed above, infants and toddlers need relatively more dietary fat than adults.

If you follow the diet plan outlined in Chapter 5, your toddler will not experience this problem. If digestive problems occur despite this dietary programme, and your child does not drink more than four to five fl. oz (230 ml) of liquid a day or no more than two glasses of juice, then the cause might well be a calcium or magnesium deficiency. If your child is constipated, give him 1 tablespoon (15 ml) of magnesium citrate each day. If, on the other hand, his bowels are loose, try a calcium–magnesium supplement.

Often, the culprit in stomach aches is a food allergy – most often milk. If your child doesn't respond to magnesium, then the nutritional detective work outlined in Chapter 4 will tell you whether this is the case with your toddler.

INFECTIONS

There are two common sources of infection: viruses, which cause colds, flu, measles, mumps and chicken pox; and bacteria, which cause inflammation, soreness and other symptoms in a specific part of the body such as the ear or the respiratory tract. Viruses and bacteria are very different, and the ways of treating the infections they cause are different, too. Antibiotics, for example, are useful against ear infections but useless against viral infections such as flu or measles.

COLDS AND OTHER VIRAL INFECTIONS

If your child comes down with any viral infection:
- *Don't force food on him.* Loss of appetite is normal and protective – eating less temporarily boosts the immune response.
- *Prevent dehydration.* Give him liquid every 15 to 30 minutes. A mouthful every 15-minutes will do. Orange juice diluted with water is a good choice because it provides some vitamin C.
- *Give him vitamin C,* about 500 mg every three hours. If his bowels become loose, stop giving it that day. The next day, give him 200 mg every three hours. If his bowels again become loose, stop vitamin C that day; the next day, give him 100 mg every four hours. Then give him about 500 mg a day until he's recovered.

Although some claim that megadoses of vitamin C are not utilized by the body and are just excreted in the urine, vitamin C in doses of 1000 mg a day or more has been shown to enhance immune function in normal human volunteers.[1]

• *Give vitamin A*, one tablespoon (30 ml) of cod-liver oil a day for five days. Viral infections produce a depletion of vitamin A stores in the liver that can last for several months.[2] An Australian study of well-nourished children with recurrent respiratory infections found that vitamin A supplementation significantly reduced the frequency of further infection, even though the children had normal blood levels of vitamin A.[3] Allergic children showed the most benefit. Vitamin A as retinol stimulates the killer T-cells in the blood. In addition, cod-liver oil contains omega-3 EFAs that help fight inflammation.

• *If he has liquid diarrhoea*, don't give him more than 200 mg of vitamin C a day. Don't give him any cod-liver oil. Diarrhoea causes the loss of both water and salt. To replace them, keep him off solid food and give him a mouthful of liquid every five to ten minutes. Dilute one part fruit juice with two parts water and add a pinch of salt; this will supply fluid, sodium, potassium and sugar, needed by the intestines to combat diarrhoea. For potassium and sugar, you can also feed him very ripe, mashed banana. At this age, concern about pesticide residues in bananas becomes secondary to their nutritional value in the treatment of diarrhoea.

Once the diarrhoea has stopped, give him high-magnesium foods – nuts, kasha (roasted buckwheat) or seafood – or a magnesium supplement for a week or two. Since magnesium itself is a laxative, keep the supplement dosage small – a good choice is liquid magnesium citrate: 1 teaspoon (5 ml) a day for ten days. This is a sub-laxative dose. A four- or five-year-old can manage 1 tablespoon (15 ml) a day.

• *I don't recommend paracetamol or aspirin to control fever* unless a child's temperature is 103° F (39.4° C) or greater, or he is in pain. A slight fever stimulates the immune system, but toddlers can go into convulsions if their fevers rise above 104° F (40° C).

• *I'm not impressed with antihistamines and cough medicines.* Hot water or lemon and honey is good for loosening a dry, hacking cough. Vitamin C in the doses I list above is a good decongestant.

BACTERIAL INFECTIONS

Ear infections

Among toddlers, these are the most common infections. Middle-ear infections need to be treated aggressively with antibiotics to prevent deafness and the spread of the infection elsewhere in the skull. Unfortunately, though, antibiotics kill bacteria indiscriminately, including good bacteria in the mouth and intestines. These good bacteria prevent the growth of such undesirable organisms as yeast, which, when it grows unchecked, can have some unpleasant consequences for a child:

• Yeast overgrowth can cause thrush (a throat infection) or a skin infection that looks like nappy rash.

• The child may become allergic to the intestinal yeast *Candida albicans*. *Candida* allergy can cause a wide variety of symptoms, from congestion to eczema.[4]

• A constant allergic inflammation in the intestinal tract can create digestive disturbances such as wind and a general feeling of being bloated, and abdominal pain, constipation or diarrhoea.

• A yeast allergy may lead to other food allergies. Normally, the intestines prevent potential allergens such as food proteins from spreading to the rest of the body, but a yeast-filled intestine becomes porous, allowing allergens to pass into the body. Allergies to yeasts and moulds in food may develop, including the yeast in bread and the natural yeast on fruits, nuts and seeds, on dried fruits such as raisins, and in commercial fruit juices. (The more 'natural' a food is, the more likely it is to contain yeast. If you leave a bottle of apple wine without preservatives at room temperature for 24 hours, it will begin to ferment. Its natural yeast is multiplying and converting its sugar to alcohol and vinegar.) Vinegar, as a yeast by-product, can provoke an allergic reaction in a yeast-sensitive child, as can fermented soya sauce.

Food yeasts don't grow in the body – they are not the same as *Candida*, the body yeast. But they can cause allergic reactions in yeast-sensitive children. Most cheeses, and particularly the various blue cheeses, Stilton and all hard cheeses, contain mould, and a yeast-sensitive child may react to them. Mould also grows quickly on strawberries and other fruits in the refrigerator, as well as on rotting foods in general. And moulds are found everywhere outside – in dirt and dead leaves on the ground, for instance.

• *Candida albicans* can produce toxic substances.[5] C. Orian Truss, a doctor in Alabama, has speculated that these toxins may enter the bloodstream to create disturbances in other parts of the body. He has found that, in certain people, emotional problems – such as anxiety and depression, and neurological symptoms that may be mistakenly diagnosed as multiple sclerosis – clear up when the person's yeast infection is treated.[6] (Sufferers of ME – myalgic encephalomyelitis, the so-called 'yuppies' disease' – have also found that treating themselves for *Candida* infections can, in some cases, relieve symptoms.) Truss's observations are controversial, but in my own practice, I have had such good results with his treatment methods that I consider using them on all sick children who have been given several courses of antibiotics or who have become ill after one course (seven to ten days) of antibiotics.

When I saw Fred, he had spent one-third of his young life taking antibiotics, but he had never been able to recover completely from a series of ear infections. His nose and chest were constantly congested.

Fred had been a healthy newborn and was fed breast milk and formula. At five months, he started on solid foods, and at six months, he had his first ear infection. He appeared to respond well to a course of antibiotics, but two months later, his ear became infected again, and from then on, his infection recurred every month. Tubes (grommets) in his ears slowed the rate of recurrence to every other month, but otherwise he made no improvement.

I confirmed my suspicion of *Candida* allergy by injecting a small dose of *Candida* extract into the skin of Fred's arm. This is a common technique for assessing immune response; people with normal immune responses will show a delayed reaction, developing a small red bump at the infection site within 24 to 48 hours. Fred, like other allergic people, developed an itchy red patch at the injection site in just ten minutes. Since his condition was serious, I recommended the following serious measures:

• A diet low in sugar and in foods containing yeast and moulds. This wasn't easy for Fred or his parent. He couldn't eat bread, cheese, dried fruits, commercial fruit juices or sweets of any kind. Because vinegar was also banned, he couldn't eat mustard, mayonnaise or ketchup. Instead of bread, he ate rice crackers or cream crackers. Because milk contains lactose (milk sugar), he was limited to 8 fl. oz (230 ml) a day. And because fruit contains sugar, he could have it only twice a day.

• We eliminated yeast-containing vitamins, and cut out all cereals containing malt. Malt is a product of the fermentation of grains with yeast and is a common flavouring in breakfast cereals. Fred could only eat unmalted cereals: porridge, puffed wheat and puffed rice.

• Nystatin (a medication that kills yeast) and a freeze-dried mixture of lactobacillus bacteria to build up the levels of normal, yeast-controlling bacteria in his intestinal tract were prescribed.

Within two weeks, Fred's ear congestion was practically gone. But he hated his diet and was starting to think about how to cheat on it. Since he had made so much progress, we gradually liberalized his diet, restricting only sugar.

At the same time, we began giving him supplements of EFAs, zinc and vitamins A and C. His hair and skin were somewhat dry, suggesting an EFA deficiency, so I recommended 1 tablespoon (30 ml) of linseed oil every day.

Fred's blood level of vitamin A was a bit low, and his hair zinc level was low as well. I recommended a yeast-free, hypoallergenic multivitamin and mineral supplement that would supply 10 mg of zinc and 5000 international units of vitamin A a day. The preparation also contained enough selenium, copper, iron and manganese to offset the potential depleting effects of a zinc supplement on these minerals.

Because vitamin C has an anti-allergic and, sometimes, even an immune-system-stimulating effect, I recommend 1000 mg of chewable vitamin C a day.

Over the next several months, Fred's ear infections gradually stopped and his congestion completely disappeared. He became more energetic and generally showed a great deal more vitality.

When your toddler has an ear infection, I recommend that you take the following steps:
- Don't push food on him. Let him eat at his own pace.
- Give him liquids frequently – follow the method described above for colds.
- Continue giving him his usual doses of linseed oil and vitamin C.
- Use paracetamol (e.g. Calpol) or aspirin for pain, not for fever.
- Use the prescribed antibiotic.
- Ask your doctor to prescribe nystatin suspension – 500,000 international units to be taken three times a day as long as your child is on the antibiotic, and for one week after.
- Give your child *Lactobacillus acidophilus* and *Lactobacillus bifidus*, both of which combat yeast. I recommend ½ teaspoon (2.5 ml) of each twice a day while your child is infected, and for one to two weeks after any course of antibiotics. (It is best to give these to your child as supplements, as commercial yoghurt may not be an adequate source of *Lactobacillus* – by the time you buy it, most of the active yoghurt culture may have died. As a test, try using a spoonful of commercial yoghurt as a starter to make homemade yoghurt; if it doesn't work, the bacteria are dead.)

Acidophilus milk does supply some active bacteria, but I prefer powdered, freeze-dried *Lactobacillus*. Be careful about what you buy; some commercial *Lactobacillus* products are worthless – they contain almost no viable organisms.

You can mix freeze-dried *acidophilus* and *bifidus* into milk, yoghurt or other food. These preparations are particularly effective against antibiotic-induced diarrhoea.

Two other yeast-controlling preparations – garlic oil and caprylic acid – aren't really suitable for toddlers. Garlic oil is quite strong in taste and smell (the deodorized product doesn't work) and you need to take a lot of it. Caprylic acid, a derivative of coconut oil, can be irritating and should be taken only in pill form. Toddlers generally aren't ready to swallow pills.

RESPIRATORY-TRACT INFECTIONS

I've found the following approach generally effective for *recurrent* or *chronic* respiratory-tract infections.

• Follow my basic meal plan for optimal nutrition to the letter.

• Your child probably has one or more nutritional deficiencies; most common are omega-3 EFA, vitamins A, C and B_6 zinc and/or iron deficiency. Give him the following:

EFAs (linseed oil)	1 tbsp (15 ml) daily
Vitamin A (cod-liver oil)	1 tsp (5 ml) daily
Vitamin C (chewable)	
Ages 1–3	500 mg a day
Ages 3–5	1000 mg a day
Vitamin B_6	25 mg a day in a chewable B complex
Zinc (dark turkey meat)	Twice a week
Iron (calf's liver)	Once or twice a week

• Search for allergies by following the directions on page 69. If a child has had lots of antibiotics, an allergy to the body yeast *Candida albicans* is likely. If your child hasn't had any antibiotics, he is most likely to be allergic to milk, wheat or house dust. A serious yeast problem usually requires treatment by a doctor who knows how to treat it effectively.

In addition, you can follow the suggestions in the previous section on how to provide your toddler with a diet free of sugar, yeast and mould. And give your child ½ teaspoon (2.5 ml) each of *Lactobacillus acidophilus* and *Lactobacillus bifidus* (*see* above, under 'Ear infections') twice a day during the infection, and for two weeks after any course of antibiotics.

ALLERGIES

ASTHMA AND ECZEMA

These allergic problems can be devastating to toddlers. Their symptoms can also be misleading. Some children with chronic coughs may actually have asthma, even though they don't wheeze or have a problem with shortness of breath. Your first step in treatment is to follow the instructions in Chapter 4 (p. 69) for evaluating your child's diet for food allergies, paying special attention to foods containing milk, yeast and moulds. (*See* pp. 105–106 under 'Ear infections' for a description of foods containing yeast and moulds.)

In allergies, as in recurrent infections, deficiencies in certain nutrients contribute to a malfunction of the immune system. One of the main problems is likely to be EFAs, which are crucial to the production of the prostaglandins that regulate all immune functioning. For omega-3s, give your child 1 tablespoon (15 ml) of linseed oil a day. You can start this right away and continue it as you go through your allergy-detection work.

Your child is likely to have a problem with omega-6 EFAs that involves more than just a dietary deficiency. In fact, back in 1931, the American paediatrician Arild Hansen found that children with eczema had abnormal levels of some omega-6 EFAs in their blood. His work attracted some attention until cortisone became available for the treatment of allergic symptoms, at which point it was ignored. But cortisone can produce terrible side-effects, such as diabetes, high blood pressure, brittle bones and atrophy of the skin. In 1981, two British dermatologists replicated Hansen's results and found that evening primrose oil was effective in relieving a group of severely afflicted patients.[7]

Evening primrose and blackcurrant oils, as we have seen, contain GLA, an EFA that is created in the body as an intermediate step in the production of prostaglandins. Every step of the prostaglandin production process is controlled by enzymes. A key enzyme in converting the main omega-6 EFA, linoleic acid (LA), into GLA is D-6-D; I call it the *Delta Force*. In children and adults with allergic eczema, asthma and hay fever, the Delta Force appears to be much less active than normal. As a result, prostaglandin production is short-circuited.

Primrose oil is sold in 250- and 500-mg capsules; I recommend Efamol brand. (Beware of products masquerading as primrose oil; they contain little or no GLA. Stick with Efamol brand.) If primrose oil is unavailable, you may use blackcurrant seed oil, also a good source of GLA. Although both oils are expensive, you need only use a small amount.

Start your toddler on two 500-mg capsules of primrose oil a day; since he probably isn't ready to swallow them, the best thing is to cut them open and rub the oil on his skin, which will absorb it into his body. Blackcurrant seed oil capsules contain as much as or more GLA than primrose oil; you can rub the oil from one of these into your child's skin each day. If he doesn't improve, increase the dose by one capsule, up to four a day.

A less effective, but also less expensive, alternative to evening primrose oil or blackcurrant oil is to provide a lot of LA so that at least some of it will be converted to GLA. If you choose this method, give your child 1 to 3 tablespoons (15–45 ml) of safflower or sunflower oil a day.

A child with omega-6 conversion problems may also have a deficiency in the co-factor vitamins and minerals that are essential in helping the Delta Force do its work of converting LA to prostaglandins. Vitamins A, certain B vitamins, magnesium, zinc and iron are particularly important. (Food sources of the co-factor minerals were listed in Chapter 4.) Unfortunately, though, food allergies may make it difficult for your child to get enough of these vitamins and minerals in his diet. The answer to this problem, of course, is supplements:

SUPPLEMENT	DOSAGE
Vitamin A (cod-liver oil)	1 tsp (5 mg) daily
Vitamins B_2 (riboflavin), B_3 (nicotinic acid) and B_6 (pyridoxine): a hypoallergenic B-complex, free of sugar, starch, yeast and artificial colouring	Should supply 25 mg of vitamin B_6 daily
Zinc (lozenge)	10 mg of zinc daily
Iron (ferrous sulphate liquid)	15 mg of iron daily
Magnesium	6 mg per pound of weight daily: 240 mg for a 40-lb child
Magnesium citrate liquid	About 1 tbsp (15 ml)
Milk of magnesia	About 1½ tsp (7.5 ml) daily

Magnesium is hard to find in a form suitable for young children. Magnesium citrate, a widely used laxative, seems to be absorbed best; to prevent a laxative effect, I have recommended a sub-laxative dose. Milk of magnesia, containing magnesium hydroxide, is second-best.

In addition to being a co-factor mineral, magnesium is an antihistamine. Histamine is a natural chemical that, when released into the blood as part of an allergic reaction, causes many of the symptoms of allergy. Animal studies have shown that magnesium deficiency increases the amount of histamine released. Magnesium has not been extensively studied in relation to childhood asthma or eczema, but some adults with magnesium deficiency show high levels of histamine which decrease when they take magnesium. And young adults with asthma have lower levels of magnesium in their blood than their non-asthmatic peers. The most common drugs used in controlling allergy symptoms are the antihistamines – magnesium may work nearly as well.

Vitamin C in high doses is also an effective antihistamine. The doses that can produce this effect – 500 to 5000 mg a day – are quite safe, even for toddlers, and vitamin C comes in chewable tablets. The main side effect of an excess of either magnesium or vitamin C is diarrhoea, which will stop when the dosage is reduced.

Maria is a good example of the successful nutritional treatment of eczema. When I first saw her, she was a sad 3½-year-old. Her parents both had allergies: her mother, asthma; her father, hay fever. As a baby, Maria was fed a milk-based formula. Her eczema started at three months. It improved when she was switched to a soya-based formula, but the minute she began eating solid foods, it returned.

Maria's doctor prescribed a cortisone cream to control her eczema, but when I saw her, she still had red, itchy, scaling patches on her chest, arms and legs. And even where there was no eczema, her skin was dry.

I recommended that her parents rub two capsules a day of evening primrose oil directly on her eczema. This reduced the symptoms enough so that the cortisone cream was applied three times a week instead of three times a day.

Since Maria's skin was still dry, I decided that she probably needed extra omega-3 EFAs as well. (The Delta Force is also crucial to the conversion of the key omega-3 EFA, LNA, to prostaglandins. In fact, Hansen successfully used linseed oil to treat eczema in his child patients.) I had her parents give her 1 tablespoon (15 ml) a day of linseed oil in juice, plus 1 teaspoon (5 ml) of mint-flavoured cod-liver oil. Over the next several weeks, her skin and hair became more lustrous and her eczema continued to improve.

I also recommended supplements of some co-factor minerals and vitamins: a zinc lozenge supplying 10 mg a day, magnesium citrate supplying 200 mg a day, a chewable multivitamin supplying B vitamins, and a chewable vitamin C supplying 500 mg a day. The magnesium and vitamin C worked as antihistamines as well as co-factors.

Because Maria was on a milk-free diet, I had her parents give her 600 mg of chewable calcium carbonate a day with her meals.

For other children with eczema, I've had to advise elimination diets, allergy desensitization and treatment for *Candida albicans* problems. Maria was lucky; she responded to EFA and co-factor nutrients, plus calcium.

BEHAVIOURAL PROBLEMS

Toddlers and pre-school children can develop all the behavioural problems common in school-age children: they can be hyperactive, prone to temper tantrums and moody. (As we saw in Chapter 4, these types of behaviour can become evident while a child is still an infant.) While such behaviour may not be as big a problem at this stage as it will be in school, it's a good idea to identify and treat the symptoms now. In my practice, I have treated many difficult children, and I've found that, with nutritional treatment, the personalities of difficult pre-schoolers often change amazingly for the better. Once a child is over seven years old, though, and patterns of aggressive, manipulative or self-destructive behaviour are well established, nutritional treatment may no longer be enough.

A child who is difficult and behaves badly creates an unhappy situation for himself. His attitudes and actions produce negative feedback that, in turn, can make his behaviour worse. He develops a poor self-image that is likely to be reinforced in school by teachers who find him hard to handle. In his excellent book *The Difficult Child*, Dr Stanley Turecki describes the difficult child as very active, easily distracted, poor at adapting to new situations, irregular in his patterns of sleeping and eating, moody and very sensitive to such external stimuli as noise, smells and bright lights. Turecki points out that some children show only some of these traits, while others are figuratively 'parent killers'.

Hyperactivity and *attention-deficit disorder* are the most common labels applied to these children's symptoms, but as diagnoses they are really spurious. Hyperactivity is not a disease; it is merely a description of the behaviour of some types of difficult children. In the pages that follow, I may use the terms *hyperactive* and *difficult* interchangeably when referring to children with all or some of the traits listed by Dr Turecki. He has outlined a behavioural programme for treating such children, but at the toddler age, a nutritional programme may be even more effective. Irritable, distractible, hypersensitive toddlers are not just poorly buffered psychologically; they are also poorly buffered biochemically. That means that they respond excessively to minor changes in their body's physiological state. They are often hypersensitive to foods and to nutritional supplements. Sometimes they are truly allergic, but often their hypersensitivities are biochemical.

Difficult children tend to eat more sugar than other children, and their parents often notice that the youngsters' behaviour deteriorates after they've eaten sweets. Whether sugar alone causes this is a matter of controversy, though. In tests at the National Institutes of Health in the United States, sugar-sensitive children who were given sugared water didn't become hyperactive or irritable, suggesting that some other factor must be at work.

A genetic factor is undoubtedly involved. Difficult children often have a parent who was or is hyperactive, restless or extremely moody. In addition, a family history of alcoholism is more common among children diagnosed as hyperactive than among other children.

Dr Ben Feingold, a California paediatrician, found that some hyperactive children are biochemically hypersensitive to salicylates, aspirin-like substances in foods and food dyes. This is not a true allergy; rather, the nervous system is sensitive to exposure to salicylates. A National Institutes of Health panel concluded that only a small fraction of hyperactive children were hypersensitive to salicylates but thought the frequency of salicylate sensitivity was great enough to warrant a trial of a low-salicylate diet in selected cases.[8] Recent data suggest that the Feingold diet may not be restrictive enough and that continued salicylate consumption even on a reduced scale may impair its effectiveness.

Almonds and other nuts, as well as apples and citrus fruits, all contain natural salicylates. Salicylates are especially concentrated in dried fruits. Many food additives, particularly artificial food colouring and such preservatives as BHT (E321), are salicylates. My experience is that artificial salicylates (food dyes and preservatives) tend to cause more problems than do natural salicylates, and that the consumption of sugar with salicylates causes a more intense response; this has been noted by others as well.[9] I have found the following measures helpful with difficult, temperamental, hyperactive, impulsive toddlers.

● Keep sugar, sweets, ice cream, cake and other high-sugar foods out of your child's diet altogether. Don't keep any in the house and ask relatives and friends not to offer them. Also limit foods high in natural sugar: don't serve him any dried fruits. Limit him to 4 fl. oz (115 ml) of fruit juice and two pieces of fresh fruit a day. Don't serve artificially coloured, flavoured, or preserved food.

● Follow the diet plan in Chapter 5 and the recipes in Chapter 10. But keep in mind that children with behavioural problems often have very irregular rhythms. They may not eat three meals a day, and they may awaken earlier and go to sleep later than other children. Give your child frequent snacks of high-protein foods such as carrot sticks with nut butter, or cream crackers with nut butter or cheese.

● EFA supplements may have a calming effect. If you are following the child's diet plan outlined in Chapter 5, you are already giving your child 1 tablespoon (15 ml) of linseed oil (or substitute 1 teaspoon/5 ml of cod-liver oil or 2 tablespoons/30 ml of walnut oil) a day to supply omega-3 EFAs. If you haven't started, start now, and pay attention to your child's behaviour, his sleep patterns and the dryness of his skin. Notice how thirsty he is. Children who are restless, have dry skins and are excessively thirsty are likely to benefit from the right EFA supplement, and you should notice some positive change within two weeks of starting linseed oil or its substitutes.

However, difficult children can be biochemically unpredictable, with strange or even negative responses to nutritional supplements. If your difficult child's skin seems to become drier with linseed oil or its substitutes, or if he becomes thirstier, stop the linseed oil and substitute 1 tablespoon (15 ml) of safflower oil. Or rub two 500-mg capsules (1 gram) of primrose oil or two 250 mg capsules of blackcurrant seed oil into his skin each day. Or keep giving him linseed oil or cod-liver or walnut oil in its place and rub two to three 500-mg capsules of primrose or blackcurrant seed oil into his skin daily. If he becomes thirstier after starting this programme, or if his skin becomes drier or his behaviour deteriorates in any way, discontinue it. In my experience, about 80 per cent of hyperactive children benefit from EFAs, with equal numbers responding to linseed oil and to primrose or blackcurrant seed oil.

Georgia, for instance, drove her parents crazy. She could act like an angel, then, for no good reason, throw a terrible temper tantrum. When I examined her, I found small rough patches on her cheeks where the skin was covered with tiny bumps. On the soles of her feet, her skin peeled. All these symptoms stopped when I put her on the child's diet plan with linseed oil.

Deborah was harder to deal with. She was a wild child, with violent mood swings – a toddler Jekyll and Hyde. She turned her bed upside down every night, had a voracious appetite and was constantly thirsty. The child's diet plan with linseed oil seemed to have no effect on these symptoms. I suggested that her mother rub three 500-mg capsules a day of primrose oil into her skin. Within 48 hours Deborah's thirst had diminished; within a week, her appetite and sleep patterns had become more normal. She remained wild, but with love and patience (fatty acids can't do everything), she became more stable as she grew into school age.

● Difficult children need more magnesium and calcium than other children. Possibly, they excrete more magnesium because of their constantly high adrenalin levels. Whatever the mechanism, their magnesium deficit in turn lowers their blood calcium levels. The two deficits lead to twitchiness, insomnia and abdominal pain.

Snacks of nuts and nut butters are a good way to provide magnesium and stabilize blood sugar. Don't give your child too much milk or cottage cheese to supply calcium; an excess of calcium and vitamin D will actually increase the amount of magnesium he needs. Limit dairy products of 16 fl. oz (460 ml) a day.

You can try one of the magnesium supplements described on page 110, 6 mg per pound of his body weight every day. If he drinks very little milk, add about 500 mg of calcium a day. If he has a problem with sleep, try giving him the magnesium at bedtime; it should have a calming effect.

● B-vitamins are tricky for this group. Although scientists don't yet know why, vitamin B supplements, including ordinary multivitamins, can actually increase a child's behaviour problems. If your child is taking a multivitamin, stop it for two weeks to see whether he becomes less jittery and aggressive or sleeps better. Sometimes individual B-vitamins, usually B_6 (pyridoxine) or B_1 (thiamin), are helpful. Try 10 mg a day of vitamin B_6 or vitamin B_1 alone, then add a B complex.

● Lead, in higher than average levels in the blood, can be associated with hyperactivity. This is most often found in poorer inner-city neighbourhoods, but recently high lead levels have also been found in middle-class American children living in older homes or blocks of flats with pipes whose joints have been soldered with lead.[10] It has been recommended that cold-water taps be run for three minutes or more each morning to clear the pipes of lead leached in overnight, and that water from the hot-water tap, which may have been sitting in an immersion heater for hours, should never be drunk or used in cooking (if your water is heated by an 'instant heat' boiler, this advice can be ignored). Iron or zinc deficiency or a diet low in calcium increases a child's susceptibility to lead poisoning.

● Allergies contribute to a wide variety of behavioural disturbances in children – about 70 per cent of hyperactive children are allergic to some kinds of food and inhalants (the pollen, dust and mould that are inhaled along with air when we breathe). Allergies may just make the child uncomfortable and irritable, but in some cases, they seem to directly affect the brain, possibly producing localized swelling or chemicals that affect brain function.

Controlled studies have shown that food allergies play a significant role in hyperactivity.[11] In a Texas study, 12 severely hyperactive children who had not responded to any therapy were tested with a sophisticated procedure called the Brain Stem Evoked Potential (BSEP). They all had abnormal electrical activity in their brains. After trials were conducted to discover the foods to which they were allergic and they stopped eating them, their BSEPs became normal and their behaviour improved.[12]

I would recommend a food trial to find out to which food or foods your child is allergic. Usually a child is allergic to several different foods, but the most common single culprit is milk. Sometimes, the 'allergy' turns out to be a hypersensitivity to salicylates, as Dr Feingold described.

If a hyperactive child has been given a lot of antibiotics, he almost always has a problem with yeast. Anti-yeast treatment has resulted in dramatic improvements in children whose behaviour has deteriorated after a course of antibiotics.

For instance, Bobby and his twin brother were healthy at birth after a normal, full-term pregnancy, but they were hard to handle, and they both seemed to have allergies. Their main symptom was chronic nasal congestion, but Bobby also developed a series of ear infections that were treated with several different antibiotics.

As the two boys entered the 'terrible twos', they drove their mother, a registered nurse, to distraction. However, the doctor felt that the boys' problems were simply expressions of their personalities.

When the twins turned three, Bobby's behaviour deteriorated, while his brother's improved. Bobby was aggressive and moody; he bit, kicked and cried easily. He was a restless sleeper and a poor eater and was very easily frightened. He was also impulsive and easily distracted. In short, he became a holy terror. His doctor suggested the drug Ritalin (methylphenidate), then frequently prescribed for hyperactive children (it has subsequently been withdrawn in the UK), but recommended waiting until Bobby was in school.

Bobby's mother suggested taking him to the Gesell Institute for an evaluation. The doctor scoffed, but she did bring the child in and I saw him. (In the US, patients do not need to be referred to consultants by their family doctors.) Bobby's antibiotic history was so strong, and was so clearly the difference between him and his twin, that I recommended six months of a yeast-free diet and a two-month course of nystatin treatment. Bobby's mother had already eliminated sugar from his diet. Now she cut out cheese, yeast breads and biscuits, vitamins made from yeast, unpeeled fresh fruit, dried fruit and commercial fruit juices. She prepared her own yeast-free bread and fresh orange juice.

After six weeks, Bobby was like a new child. Everyone – his parents, his relatives, even his family doctor – recognized the changes in his personality. (For more on yeasts, and a yeast-free diet, see Chapter 7.)

Andy, though, was a little boy with a more serious problem – in fact, he may never completely recover. At two, Andy was diagnosed as *autistic*, meaning that he did not communicate with the outside world. Some children appear to be autistic almost from birth. Others, like Andy, appear to be normal at first. By two, Andy had begun to speak. Then he had a series of respiratory infections, for which he was given antibiotics. Within a few weeks after his second ear infection, he stopped talking. He became much less responsive, and would grow violent if he were thwarted in any way. His appetite became voracious. His parents took him to a series of specialists, one of whom eventually diagnosed him as autistic.

Andy's parents chose a programme of calculated permissiveness: They wouldn't force him to do anything. Instead they would try to shape his world to conform to him. They brought in mother's helpers and volunteers to cater to him.

Slowly, Andy became less difficult and more predictable. But when, at three, he was given another round of antibiotics for an ear infection, he completely regressed and lost all self-control. He had seizure-like falling spells and developed chronic diarrhoea.

A friend of Andy's mother who was being treated for a yeast-allergy problem suggested that Andy might have a similar allergy. His mother took him to a clinical ecologist, a doctor specializing in allergies and other hypersensitive reactions to the environment. This doctor skin-tested Andy and told his mother that he had multiple food allergies. He suggested that she stop giving Andy any food and substitute Vivonex, a hyoallergenic but sugar-containing food substitute. At first, Andy's behaviour improved; he seemed more 'of this world'. But then he regressed again. At that point, his mother brought him to me.

My assessment was that antibiotics were the main cause of Andy's problems. By killing off the good bacteria in his intestines, the antibiotics had allowed an overgrowth of yeast that had damaged the intestinal lining, creating multiple food allergies. I also thought that the yeast overgrowth might have had a toxic effect on Andy's body, leading to biochemical disturbances that could account for some of his behaviour.

I had Andy stop Vivonex and start eating seafood and vegetables. We experimented with several diets and found that he did best on rice, vegetables, tofu and some fish. We also tried various drugs to decrease the yeast in his intestines. Andy reacted poorly to most of them, but he was able to tolerate an over-the-counter coconut-oil derivative (unavailable in the UK). We added two *Lactobacillus* preparations: an *acidophilus* and a *bifidus*.

Andy also had an extensive metabolic evaluation that uncovered a problem in digestion – undigested fat and starch were present in his stool. He had deficiencies of vitamins A and B_6, and magnesium, copper, zinc, iron and selenium. He couldn't tolerate a B-vitamin supplement; it made him more aggressive and interfered with his sleep. But he did well with supplements of magnesium, cod-liver oil, linseed oil, primrose oil, zinc, copper, selenium and iron. When he stopped these, he withdrew and began falling apart again.

When I first saw Andy, his face had a dull expression, his tongue lolled out of his mouth and he had dark puffy rings around his eyes. He couldn't walk by himself. After a year of intense treatment, he had become affectionate and expressive and could walk and run. From a distance, he looked quite normal, although he still didn't talk. Best of all, though, a repeat psychological assessment indicated that *Andy isn't autistic*. His ability to learn is excellent, and he has now begun to speak.

Few children have problems as extreme as Andy's, but his story underlines the importance of the points I've been stressing in this chapter.

● *Antibiotics can have a devastating effect on some children.*
● *A yeast infection can create severe allergic and, possibly, biochemical disturbances.*

I feel strongly that all children who take antibiotics should be given treatment to normalize their intestinal flora. This includes a low-sugar, high-fibre diet and both *Lactobacillus acidophilus* and *Lactobacillus bifidus* preparations. If the child is given antibiotics again, or if he's allergic to start with, I recommend nystatin to inhibit yeast growth.

Finally, the stories of Andy and the other children I've told in this chapter also underline my experiences that even the most severe behavioural disturbances in children may respond to nutritional treatment.

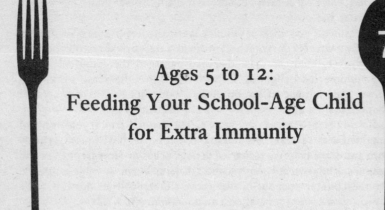

Ages 5 to 12:
Feeding Your School-Age Child
for Extra Immunity

The school-age child is moving out beyond her home, and this means new experiences. At school, your child will encounter a new, more disciplined environment that even a day-care centre or nursery school may not have prepared her for. New stresses will become part of her life – she'll face pressures to learn, to compete and to conform to unfamiliar rules. Stress will test her immune system, and so will the barrage of new viruses and bacteria she will encounter, especially if she hasn't spent time in a nursery school or day-care centre. But the foods you feed her, and the eating habits you reinforce, can keep her a vibrantly healthy child whose body is well able to cope with new challenges.

Eating habits are especially important at this age because, for the first time, she will have to cope on her own with other people's eating patterns and that modern menace, junk food. In her pre-school years, it was relatively easy to control her access to junk food, although she was certainly exposed to it on TV and on outings with other parents. Now, she's on her own much more. She will eat and sleep at friends' houses, and discover that other kids eat sweets and ice cream, sticky buns and fairy cakes – not to mention crisps – at home. She may also find they eat fried foods, or a lot of meat. Perhaps for the first time, she will question your menus.

How do you cope?

By following the sensible basic nutrition plan in this chapter, you'll keep your child's diet high in essential fatty acids (EFAs) and in the co-factor nutrients that will help her body metabolize EFAs: vitamins A, B_6 (pyridoxine), C, E and the minerals magnesium, zinc, copper and selenium. EFA metabolism, you may recall from Chapter 1, produces the prostaglandins that keep her immune system as well as her heart, lungs and nervous system working well.

She'll also have plenty of iron and a good supply of the anti-oxidants that protect her immune system as iron does its work: vitamins A, C, E, B_2 (riboflavin) and B_3 (nicotinic acid), and zinc, copper, manganese and sulphur. Anti-oxidants protect against the effects of radiation, help the body defend itself against the toxins in other environmental pollutants, and provide important protection against free radicals, which are found in heat-damaged oils used in fastfood outlets. Free radicals damage cells, including immune cells, and they turn up in chips, hamburgers, deep-fried fish and chicken nuggets – in short, in all deep-fried food, whether prepared by somebody's mother or at McDonald's.

If necessary, in addition to the linseed oil or walnut oil or cod-liver oil you'll give her every day to provide her with omega-3 EFAs, she can take supplements of vitamins C and E to provide an extra boost of anti-oxidants, or she can take magnesium to correct a deficiency that could contribute to allergies.

Away from home she's going to be exposed to all kinds of anti-nutrients – the sugar, fats, salt and phosphates that interfere with prostaglandin production and so undermine her immune system. Soft drinks and commercial pastries are loaded with sugar, but sugar also turns up in peanut butter, ketchup and other spreads and condiments, and in such luncheon meats as turkey roll. Fats – especially hydrogenated or partially hydrogenated oils – are added to commercial baked goods, sauces, luncheon meats and virtually all manufactured snacks and foods. Hydrogenation destroys the essential fatty acids in otherwise healthy oils. Fats and sugar, which provide neither vitamins nor minerals, are major causes of obesity. And they may increase the body's need for certain nutrients to help it undo the damage they do.

Manufactured foods are also usually very high in salt. Check the label on a can of soup – it may contain almost 1000 mg of sodium, as much as your child should consume in the entire day. Canned or bottled spaghetti sauces – almost any food in a can or bottle, for that matter – many breakfast cereals, most snack foods, luncheon meats and cheeses, and many baked goods have salt added. Yet children already get all the salt they need from foods in which it occurs naturally. Added salt only contributes to the possibility of high blood pressure, while depleting the body's supplies of magnesium by triggering its excretion into the urine.

When your child consumes most soft drinks, she'll be taking in phosphates, chemicals added to balance the carbonation. Phosphates are also widely used as preservatives in manufactured food. Wherever they're used, they block her body's ability to absorb calcium and magnesium from the nutritious food she eats at home.

But take heart: you can still control *most* of the food she eats, including her school lunches. If her basic diet is sound, a little junk food once in a while won't hurt. And, if she's used to a low-fat, low-sugar diet, she's not likely to crave high-sugar sweets or deep-fried chicken nuggets. She may very well find them too sweet, too greasy. When the kids go to the local Pizza Hut, she might even fix a salad at the salad bar. I'll help you develop a strategy to use on the days when she comes home from a friend's house and says, 'Sally's mum lets her have chips and Coke every afternoon!'

WHAT TO FEED YOUR SCHOOL-AGE CHILD

Nutritional needs don't change much at this age. To ensure normal growth, a healthy immune system and optimum intellectual development, she will still need a balanced, varied diet of foods low in sugar and fat and high in vitamins, minerals and essential fatty acids. She should have three meals and a snack every day.

- a high-protein breakfast
- a packed lunch you prepare at home
- an after-school snack
- a nutritious dinner

BREAKFAST

Never skip breakfast. Your child should get at least one-third of the nutrients she needs every day from this meal, and it should be high in protein, not carbohydrates. Protein lowers the levels of a brain chemical called serotonin, which plays a role in making people sleepy. Most children respond to a high-protein breakfast by remaining alert all morning long. A high-carbohydrate breakfast, on the other hand, makes them (and you) drowsy because it enhances the brain's synthesis of serotonin. It's worth getting up 15 minutes earlier so that you'll have enough time to fix a good breakfast.

Protein

Eggs are a good source of protein, but serve them boiled (for at least eight minutes). Don't fry or scramble them; this oxidizes the cholesterol in the egg yolk, producing chemicals that damage blood vessels. Boiled eggs are delicious on wholewheat toast.

Tofu has no cholesterol, so you can stir-fry it or scramble it. It's a good breakfast food, and this is a good time to introduce your child to it. (*See* Chapter 10.)

Homemade cereal provides protein and many vitamins and minerals; homemade porridge, muesli, and Swiss muesli are all delicious. (*See* Chapter 10.)

Seeds and nuts help raise the protein and mineral content of cereals; you'll use them in muesli, but you can also mix them into porridge or any sugar-free commercial cereal. (Check the child's breakfast menus in Chapter 5 for tips on these and other breakfast choices such as sesame waffles, that your child will still enjoy. Also, check the information on pp. 91–92 on convenience foods.)

Leftovers can be good sources of protein, although some people don't like fish or beans for breakfast.

Milk provides protein and calcium. (*Note:* Your child doesn't need to drink whole milk any longer. It's time to serve her low-fat milk and yoghurt, if she'll take them.)

Definitely avoid bacon! This traditional breakfast staple has too much fat, salt and cancer-causing nitrates. Ditto ham and sausage.

Vitamin C

Fresh fruit and orange or grapefruit juice are important sources of vitamin C and should be part of every breakfast. Fresh fruit makes cereals deliciously sweet.

Carbohydrates

Carbohydrates should not be the main part of breakfast because, as I said above, they create drowsiness rather than alertness. But as an adjunct to high-protein foods, 100 per cent wholewheat bread or toast is delicious. Check the label to make sure *whole* wheat flour is the first ingredient listed (stone-ground wholewheat flour is best). *Wheat flour* is just a euphemism for refined white flour; *unbleached flour* is highly refined. Avoid them. The wheat can also be sprouted or cracked. Other whole grains, such as rye, barley and maize, make excellent ingredients. A crunchy, multigrain bread makes terrific toast.

Serve toast either topped by an egg, or with stir-fried or scrambled tofu, or with nut butter, sugar-free apple and pear spread, or sugar-free fruit conserve. Don't use butter or margarine – the first is pure fat, the second pure hydrogenated fat. Naturally, you won't serve commercial buns, muffins, coffee cake or pastries.

At eight, Justin was eating a soft roll and glass of orange juice for breakfast. By lunchtime, he was famished and ate everything on the school lunch menu, including dessert. He wasn't doing well in school; he was inattentive and sleepy and didn't read well. Since he perked up for playtime, his teacher thought he was just not motivated to learn. At night, though, it was a different story – Justin was rambunctious and lively. He had a hard time falling asleep.

It was obvious to me that Justin's body rhythms were out of sync with his world. My solution was to put him on a high-protein breakfast of egg, tofu, meat, milk, yoghurt or cottage cheese. Most carbohydrates – pasta, whole-grain bread, vegetables and fruits – were shifted to dinner, when he ate no meat.

I also had Justin's parents cut out TV at night and begin to structure the time in ways that would help him settle down to a good night's sleep. In addition to a family meal, Justin's homework and a warm bath, they began giving him ten minutes or more of undivided attention every night.

Within two weeks, Justin became more alert in school. His reading – and his marks – improved. And he slept better at night.

Sharing time with your children is an important way of expressing love, that all-important 'invisible nutrient' children need. There is no age limit on the need for people who love each other to spend time together; your child will need this special time-sharing until he's at least 18 – and perhaps older.

Is there always enough time to give your child some undivided attention? Yes. If you think about how to spend the time that's available, rather than worry about how little time you have, you'll find there is time even if you have several children. The parents of three boys gave each boy 10 or 20 minutes of 'exclusive private time' every day. Each boy was allowed to say how he wanted this spent: sharing dinner preparations, playing, reading, a brisk walk or a quiet conversation. *Time* is the most previous gift we can give to those we love.

Fibre

At this age, fibre becomes important because your child can get it only from her food, and breakfast is a good meal at which to provide it. (Youngsters under five can't tolerate fibre well, so I haven't recommended it before.) Fibre feeds the good bacteria in the intestine that keep yeast from getting out of hand (*see* pp. 72–73 for a thorough discussion of what yeast can do when it gets out of hand). Fibre also helps prevent bowel cancer and also appears to help prevent heart disease later in life.

What is fibre? Simply stated, it's the part of plants that isn't digested by enzymes in the stomach and intestines. It comes in two varieties: *soluble* and *insoluble*. Insoluble fibre doesn't even dissolve in powerful stomach acid. It is coarse and has the effect of scrubbing the intestine, helping to prevent bowel cancer. Wheat bran is full of insoluble fibre.

Soluble fibre does dissolve in digestive juices to form a soft gel. Your child doesn't digest it but the good bacteria in her intestine do; it supports their growth. This bacterial digestion of soluble fibre releases substances that can lower cholesterol, smooth the absorption of sugar, kill harmful bacteria and yeasts and nourish the large intestine.

Fruits, pulses and oat bran all contain soluble fibre – oat bran is the best source. The typical Western diet doesn't supply enough fibre, so it's vital that you serve fibre-rich foods. Just make sure that you give your child a lot of water to drink whenever you serve her a high-fibre food. Without water to dilute it, fibre can actually be constipating. Children who have frequent or chronic abdominal pain, with or without accompanying constipation, often benefit from a high-fibre diet.

When eight-year-old Sally's doctor sent her to me, she complained every day of stomach aches. She moved her bowels every other day, and her stools were hard.

Since the doctor could find no physical cause for Sally's abdominal pains, he put them down to anxiety and stress. Sally's diet was better than most, but far from perfect: she ate a lot of chicken and fish, salads, eggs, yoghurt, cheese, bananas and fruit juices. Although low in sugar and high in nutrients, this diet provided few foods rich in fibre.

I asked her mother to substitute fresh fruits, such as apples and berries, for fruit juice, and add whole grains to her diet, substituting brown rice and wholewheat bread for white rice and bread. She ate more pulses (beans, lentils, chickpeas, etc.), especially in salads. (Most basic salad ingredients – e.g. lettuce, cucumbers, celery – are 99 per cent water, and, therefore, very low in fibre.) She also ate pulses as a protein substitute for meat. For breakfast, she began eating porridge with added oat bran and fresh fruit.

Within three weeks, Sally's abdominal pains had stopped, and she was having normal daily bowel movements.

I could have treated Sally with psyllium husks (the basis for Metamucil, used for 'regularity' by many older adults) to provide fibre, but whenever possible it's better to change a child's eating habits to prevent her problems from recurring rather than simply to dose her with unnecessary supplements.

The most necessary supplement is linseed oil; breakfast is the ideal time to give your child the 1 tablespoon (15 ml) of linseed oil that most children continue to need each day. Mix it into her cereal or juice, or give it to her straight. (Keep this oil in the refrigerator after you've opened it.) You may substitute 1 teaspoon (5 ml) of cod-liver oil or 2 tablespoons (30 ml) of walnut oil if linseed oil is unavailable.

LUNCH

Can you trust the lunch served at your child's school? Unless she goes to a special school indeed, the odds are you can't. Even when schools try to serve 'balanced meals' that include vegetables, they generally contain too much sugar, fat and salt, and too little in the way of such key minerals as zinc and copper. Besides, hot school dinners sit in steam tables while the heat destroys vitamins by the minute. (The food is therefore more nutritious in the first lunch sitting than the second or third.)

You're better off making your child's lunch yourself. Sandwiches are delicious and convenient and supply a good mixture of ingredients. Whole-wheat pita (pocket) bread not only stands up under all kinds of fillings, but it is made without sugar or oil. Wholewheat bread, in addition to being 100 per cent whole wheat (see above under 'Breakfast'), should be made without preservatives or hydrogenated or partially hydrogenated oils. This eliminates all the major brands of commercial bread. Try baking your own bread or buying it from a good bakery or healthfood shop. Since fat helps make and keep bread moist, it is virtually always used – try to find bread made with unhydrogenated safflower or soya oil. Keep it fresh in the refrigerator or freezer; to restore its natural flavour, toast it lightly.

Spreads and fillers

You can fill wholewheat bread or pita pockets with plain home-cooked meat, fish or poultry; nut butter or apple and pear spread, falafel (ground chickpea balls) and hummus (see Chapter 10) with alfalfa sprouts and grated cheese; or with salmon, tuna or chicken with homemade mayonnaise and chopped celery. Keep away from commercial luncheon meats – sausage, turkey roll, ham and so forth are chock-full of fat, sugar and salt.

Spreads. Don't use commercial spreads such as ketchup or mayonnaise. In fact, no matter how many times your school-age child tells you that his friends' mothers let them use ketchup, keep it out of your kitchen altogether. It is full of sugar. (There is one exception, described in Chapter 10.)

Commercial mayonnaise is a dangerous food because it is usually made with partially hydrogenated vegetable oils as well as egg yolks (the partially hydrogenated oils are more nutritionally harmful than the 10 mg or so of cholesterol in the egg yolks). But you can get tofu-based mayonnaise in healthfood shops. It's the best commercial mayonnaise because it supplies protein and minerals and is free of destructive fats. You may also be able to find egg-yolk mayonnaise made with pure, unhydrogenated soya oil.

The best mayonnaise, though, is homemade – see Chapter 10 for both tofu and egg-yolk versions. Homemade linseed- or walnut-oil mayonnaise is a good way to get omega-3 EFAs into your family's diet. (With a food processor, it's easy to make any homemade sandwich spread or filler.)

You can get around mayonnaise altogether by making chicken sandwiches with a dressing of oil and tarragon vinegar, then mixing in just enough yoghurt to bind it together.

Commercial mustard is all right, but many children don't like it, and it's not suitable for all sandwiches. Try a mild, whole-grain mustard with cold meat or poultry, or a relatively sweet Dijon tarragon mustard with poultry or cold fish. You can also mix tarragon mustard with yoghurt and a little oil to make an interesting spread or dip. Use one part mustard to two parts yoghurt and a dash of oil, and mix well.

Fillers. This is a good way to use leftover meat, fish or poultry. For colour, taste, crunchiness and vitamins, include vegetables in the sandwich, or separately – sliced tomatoes or green peppers provide vitamins A and C, for instance.

Nut butters make excellent fillers. I'm not happy about peanut butter because of a strange quirk in the way its oils are structured. It has a tendency to raise cholesterol levels, so walnut and almond butters are preferable, although harder to find. Walnuts contain omega-3 EFAs and almonds are rich in magnesium. (*See* Chapter 10.)

If you do use peanut butter, try to buy one that is sugar-free and, if possible, salt-free. Healthfood shops usually carry at least one variety, and even some large manufacturers are producing sugar-free peanut butter.

To make nut butters, especially peanut butter, more nutritious, mix in sesame butter (tahini) and/or soya flour or ground sunflower seeds. These add protein, zinc and copper.

To make nut butters more flavourful, add apple and pear spread, chopped dates or raisins for sweetness. For taste, texture and vitamins, mix in or add to the sandwich such vegetables as shredded carrots (vitamin A), alfalfa sprouts, sliced tomatoes or sliced green peppers (vitamins A and C).

Hummus, made of mashed chick-peas and tahini, makes a good substitute for nut butter. You can use nut butter or hummus every day; for their high magnesium, serve them at least twice a week. You can add linseed oil to nut butters to make them moister.

Fish and salads. Squeeze lemon on tuna or salmon, or some sardines. Canned salmon is high in vitamin B_{12}, and sardines are high in calcium, iron and vitamin D. Both supply some omega-3 EFAs, but not enough, in the tinned form, to obviate the need for linseed or cod-liver or walnut oil. Canned tuna is rich in nicotinic acid (vitamins B_3) and other B vitamins, but read the label for its salt content. Even low-salt brands may have hidden salt; I advise rinsing all tinned fish before you use it.

Make chicken, turkey or tuna fish sandwiches with homemade mayonnaise or tofu (see Chapter 10). Add sliced tomatoes or bean sprouts. Some children like minced olives, but be sure to rinse them off.

Sweets

A piece of fresh fruit is best: send along an apple, pear, peach, quartered orange or a banana. Don't use dried fruits or oatmeal biscuits because they leave sugary deposits on the teeth.

AFTER-SCHOOL SNACKS

Children need to eat more than three times a day because they are active and growing. A healthy after-school snack can make an important contribution to your child's diet.

Milk or *yoghurt* both make excellent snack foods, although your child shouldn't need more than 16 fl. oz (460 ml) of milk a day.

Lunch sandwiches also make excellent snacks.

Homemade fast foods will be essential for variety:

• Add chopped *fresh or dried fruit* and *nuts* to plain, low-fat yoghurt.

• *Mini-pizza:* grill a wholewheat muffin with cheese and tomato; or *pocket-pizza:* fill a wholewheat pita with mozzarella and tomato, and bake for five minutes in a 350° F (180° C, gas mark 4) oven.

• *Muesli bars* (see Chapter 10 for recipe).

• *Crispbread or crisps with spread or dip.* Avoid such standard fare as potato crisps; they're loaded with heat-damaged, partially hydrogenated vegetable oils and salt, as are most crispbreads, for that matter. Choose a brand, such as the Scandinavian crispbreads, that is made without oil. If you can find commercial tacos or tortillas without added oil, they can make good crisps. Just bake the tortillas until crisp (see Chapter 10). Use nut butters on crispbread, make Mexican bean or tofu dip, or season yoghurt with dill or chopped chives. Add linseed oil to nut butters to turn them into dips, or add yoghurt to sesame butter (see Chapter 10).

• *Yoghurt or tofu smoothies* (see Chapter 10) make great snacks; you can also freeze them to make ice lollies.

• *Homemade, low-sugar, oatmeal–sesame–raisin biscuits* (see Chapter 10).

• *Frozen nut-fruit balls*, made with chopped dried fruit, nuts and seeds (see Chapter 10).

DINNER

I can't emphasize enough the importance of making this a family affair. Eat at the kitchen or dining table, and talk to each other. Don't watch TV or read. Eating should be, deliberately and consciously, a complete experience, not something you do on the run, or while doing something else. But if you don't set the example yourself, your child will never learn the pleasure of a relaxed meal in the company of loved ones.

If your child has had a high-protein breakfast, a nutritious lunch and a wholesome after-school snack, you don't need to fix a big dinner. A light supper is fine: soup, salad and bread may be all she needs.

Many families eat most of their daily protein at dinner, but as we have seen, this is a mistake, especially for children. Now is the time for carbohydrates.

Carbohydrates

Starches. Most children love mashed potatoes, but you can be more intensive than that. Serve brown rice, whole-grain breads, kasha (roasted buckwheat) or wholewheat pasta. Add kasha to cooked noodles; your child will love it.

Soups. Both hot and cold soups make excellent supper items. To chop vegetables, a food processor saves time.

Vegetables. Serve a variety of vegetables, and keep the different colours in mind for different minerals and vitamins. Try to have at least one baked or steamed green vegetable plus on orange or yellow vegetable. You can also stir-fry vegetables.

For topping, instead of using high-fat butter or margarine, squeeze a fresh lemon over your vegetables, or make my basic linseed- or walnut-oil and vinegar dressing. You can add herbs and/or minced garlic to the dressing. Grated cheddar or Parmesan cheese makes an excellent topping.

Experiment with various combinations of vegetables, or make a whole meal combining different textures and colours. That artful and versatile bean food, tofu, seems made to be stir-fried with a variety of vegetables.

Protein

Although you will be concentrating on carbohydrates, you will eat some protein at dinner-time.

Pulses. Serve beans, peas and lentils twice a week, if possible. You can combine them with pasta and sauce, rice, fish or poultry. In addition to protein, pulses provide magnesium, soluble fibre, minerals and lectins, natural chemicals that stimulate the immune response of the white blood cells in the intestines.

Seafood. Serve two or three times a week. Shellfish and scaled fish are low in saturated fats and supply omega-3 EFAs and essential minerals. My bouillabaisse recipe is a whole meal in a bowl (*see* Chapter 10).

Meat. Liver is rich in vitamin A, zinc, iron and that very important B vitamin, folic acid. Your child needs all of these nutrients to keep building a strong immune system. For that reason, I sometimes recommend eating liver at least once a week.

Beef, lamb, pork and veal are high in saturated fat, so don't serve this group more than twice a week. (If possible, get organic beef, now available from a few suppliers.) It may take a while to lose the craving for – or the habit of – eating red meat more frequently, but eventually you will find you enjoy other sources of protein.

Poultry. The best way to serve chicken or turkey is roasted. Buy a fresh small turkey or chicken from your butcher. Fresh poultry tastes better and is likely to be healthier than its battery-raised, thawed supermarket counterparts. To roast poultry, clean the cavity and rub the inside with a sliver of fresh garlic. (If you like the taste of garlic, leave two or three cloves in the cavity.) Rub the outside of the bird with fresh paprika. (Buy the best Hungarian paprika and keep it in the refrigerator.) Roast in a low-heat oven. Set the bird on a rack so that the fat drips down into the pan.

Another method for chicken is to brown it first to keep in the flavour and juices, then cook it with 8 fl. oz (230 ml) of chicken or vegetable stock for 30 minutes in a pressure cooker. This saves time and retains flavour, minerals and vitamins. However you cook poultry, though, remove the fat-loaded skin before serving.

Sweets

A sweet is traditional after dinner, but it's here that many parents' best intentions go awry. Yet desserts can be nutritious as well as delicious. I generally avoid honey – nutritionally, it's not much better than sugar. I rely on fruit for sweetness and vitamin C, yoghurt or tofu for calcium, and nuts and seeds for other minerals.

Many of the snack foods listed above – yogurt with chopped fruit, or homemade muesli bars, smoothies, oatmeal, biscuits or frozen nut balls – make excellent sweets. So do yoghurt or tofu pudding or ice lollies, low-sugar fruit-nut pies and spice cakes with optional creamy yoghurt or tofu toppings.

These are all easy to prepare, and you can make them ahead of time in batches. (*See* Chapter 10.)

Baked apples are a snap and fill the house with a wonderful aroma. In baking, some of the starch in them turns to sugar, making the apples sweeter. You can simply bake washed, cored apples for an hour in a low oven with a little cinnamon. Baste them in their own juices as they cook. If you like, add a few unsulphured raisins and a tablespoon of homemade muesli in the core cavity.

Fresh or dried fruit (preferably without preservatives) is the only preparation-free, commercially available sweet that's not loaded with anti-nutrients.

HOLIDAY AND PARTY FOOD

Any of the snacks and sweets are fine for parties. Popcorn is all right, but nutritionally limited – you can add nourishment by sprinkling hot popcorn with grated Parmesan.

Christmas is a holiday for sweet, moist, nutritious spice cakes and fruit breads, with lots of goodies mixed in. For Easter, try fruit and nut balls wrapped in coloured foil instead of jelly babies and chocolate. (*See* Chapter 10.)

Encourage your child to help prepare such holiday treats in advance; you'll both enjoy the sharing and the creative fun. (*See* other suggestions in Chapter 8.)

SUPPLEMENTS

Omega-3 essential fatty acids (EFAs) help maintain your child's immune system in top form, protect her against cancer and heart disease later in life, and ensure that her nervous system functions properly. So it is vital that you give your child omega-3s in some form every day. The easiest way is to give her 1 tablespoon (15 ml) linseed oil or 1 teaspoon (5 ml) cod-liver oil each day. She can take it straight, like medicine, just before a meal or juice, or you can mix it into her food or juice. (Drink quickly, because juice and oil soon separate.)

If you notice that your child is excessively thirsty, or if she has dry skin or dull, lifeless hair, she may have an EFA deficiency. For a full discussion of how to deal with this, see pages 12–15.

Vitamins C and E and magnesium are key supplements for a properly regulated immune system. All are completely safe. However, a healthy child following my basic meal plan needs no nutritional supplement as a rule, except for linseed oil or the substitutes for it I have suggested. If there is a strong family history of allergy, or if the child has problems with allergies, infections or behaviour, these supplements may be added to a healthy diet.

Vitamins C and E

Five hundred milligrams of vitamin C and 100 international units of vitamin E daily provide children with greater anti-oxidant protection than good food alone can give them. These two vitamins are especially indicated for children in urban or industrial areas who are exposed to considerable air pollution.[1]

Magnesium

Growing children need 6 mg of magnesium per pound of body weight every day. This amounts to about 240 mg a day for a small five-year-old and 600 mg a day for a growing twelve-year-old. These figures, calculated by the American expert Dr Mildred Seelig, executive director of the American College of Nutrition, and her European counterpart, Dr Jean Durlach, chairman of the Society for Development of Research on Magnesium, are greater than the current US RDA (there are no RDAs for magnesium in the UK). Despite this, 70 per cent of children in the United States consume less than two-thirds the RDA in their food each day, so they are getting an even smaller fraction of their real need.

Magnesium has a subtle but very important effect on a child's immune system: it is among the most important of the co-factor vitamins and minerals that help the body metabolize EFAs to make prostaglandins. Magnesium deficiency also causes the body to release more histamine, which increases the severity of allergic symptoms such as congestion, coughing and shortness of breath.

The best food sources for this important mineral are nuts, nut butters such as almond or peanut butter, seeds, vegetables and seafood.

Magnesium deficiency can also be caused by increased excretion of magnesium in the urine. High intakes of salt (sodium), sugar, fats, protein, phosphorus or vitamin D all increase magnesium excretion. So do stress and physical exercise. If your child is very athletic, she will need a plentiful supply of high-magnesium foods.

If your child is athletic and/or has been eating a typical Western diet, high in salt, sugar, fats and the other anti-nutrients, she may also need a supplement. If she has allergies, she definitely does.

Typical symptoms of mild magnesium deficiency include:

- *irritability:* restlessness, poor sleeping habits, hyperactivity
- *fatigue*
- *muscle spasm:* twitches, abdominal pain, headaches or bed-wetting

- *creepy-crawly feeling on the skin:* older children who are able to verbalize their symptoms may describe this as a pins-and-needles sensation
- *grinding the teeth at night*

If your child has any of these symptoms, you can find out whether it's caused by magnesium deficiency by a simple test: Give her an oral magnesium supplement for four weeks and see whether the symptom or symptoms improve in that time. This can be a much better way to determine magnesium deficiency than any laboratory measure now available. You will soon know if the dose is too high because your child will develop diarrhoea. If she does, just reduce the dose. (If your child has a kidney problem, consult your doctor before using any magnesium supplement. Children with kidney problems can develop too high a level of magnesium in their blood.)

When I saw six-year-old Betsy, she was a nervous child who slept poorly and was constipated. Almost every day, she complained of abdominal pain. Her reflexes were hyperactive: when I tapped the skin over her facial nerve, it twitched. (This is called Chvostek's sign.) Betsy wasn't getting much magnesium in her diet, and her symptoms suggested deficiency to me. When I prescribed three magnesium chloride tablets a day, her abdominal pains, irritability and constipation disappeared, and she began to sleep better.

Which magnesium supplement to use. Magnesium comes in a bewildering variety of forms. All magnesium (and all other mineral) supplements comprise the mineral attached to something else, such as an oxide, chloride, citrate, gluconate, orotate, aspartate, amino acid chelate. A 500 mg magnesium oxide pill contains about 200 mg magnesium and 300 mg oxide – each element weighs about the same. Magnesium orotate, on the other hand, supplies only about 30 mg of magnesium in a 500-mg pill, because the orotate makes up 470 mg. A true amino acid chelate of magnesium supplies 30 to 50 mg of magnesium in a 500-mg tablet. If it claims to supply more, it's not a true chelate; it's a mixture of magnesium oxide and amino acids, which isn't any better than plain magnesium oxide.

Magnesium oxide is safe and can be effective, but it usually comes in a big, chalky tablet that is hard to swallow. So-called amino acid chelates, including magnesium aspartate, are expensive and seldom worth the money because they usually contain primarily magnesium oxide but cost much more.

Magnesium citrate is a good magnesium source if it's given in a sub-laxative dose. (Magnesium citrate is a common laxative, but a sub-laxative dose won't have that effect.) One tablespoon (15 ml) daily of magnesium citrate can correct a magnesium deficiency for just pennies. Unfortunately, most magnesium citrate liquids contain artificial flavour, sugar and/or sorbitol. Pure magnesium citrate capsules are hard to find; ask your chemist or local healthfood shop whether they can order some for you.

Magnesium chloride is an excellent source of magnesium; the chloride enhances its absorption. A good source is enteric-coated magnesium chloride tablets – the coating decreases gastric irritation. Give your child three tablets a day. Taken at bedtime, magnesium can enhance sleep.

Not recommended. Antacids such as Maalox and Gelusil contain magnesium but they also contain aluminium, a toxic metal. Magnesium carbonate, from dolomite, is often not well-absorbed, and dolomite is often contaminated with lead.

Calcium

School-age children who dislike, or can't tolerate, dairy products tend to become calcium deficient. This can be a serious problem because it produces brittle bones, and may also produce symptoms very similar to those caused by magnesium deficiency, such as muscle spasm and irritability. In fact, calcium complements magnesium in its calming, muscle-relaxing effects.

Your child only needs about 16 fl. oz (460 ml) of milk or yoghurt a day to avoid a calcium deficiency: 8 fl. oz (230 ml) of milk supplies 288 mg; 8 fl. oz (230 ml) of yoghurt supplies 174 mg.

Other calcium-rich foods are almond butter, bean soup and tortillas. For a more complete list of calcium-rich foods, see page 83.

If your child is not eating or drinking enough milk or yoghurt every day, *and* if she's not eating lots of non-dairy calcium-rich foods such as fish with bones (tinned salmon, sardines and herring), tofu, shellfish or nuts, I recommend 600 mg of a calcium supplement daily. I don't recommend more than that amount because too much calcium interferes with vitamin D metabolism and with your child's ability to absorb zinc and iron.

Recommended forms. Calcium carbonate from oyster shells is one of the cheapest forms of calcium. It is best absorbed after being dissolved by stomach acid, so always give it to your child with food. Chewable calcium carbonate wafers, with no sugar or colouring added, are available at healthfood stores: 600 mg daily.

Calcium citrate is best if your child has allergies, because allergies are sometimes associated with a decrease in the production of the stomach acid needed before calcium carbonate can be absorbed. Give her two or three tablets a day.

Not recommended. Calcium carbonate from bone meal or dolomite, both of which can be contaminated with lead. Also to be avoided are varieties that contain sugar and talc (talc has been shown to promote tumours in animals).

Zinc

This element continues to be one of your child's most important nutrients. It is a key co-factor mineral, helping the body metabolize EFAs, and it is also an important anti-oxidant, protecting white blood cells while they protect your child. Zinc deficiency impairs immune function and predisposes a child to many different kinds of infection. It can also impair growth.

Strenuous exercise, high-protein diets and allergies increase the loss of zinc from the body. Diets too high in iron and calcium can block the body's absorption of this mineral. Mild zinc deficiency, like mild magnesium deficiency, is very hard to test. Dr Ananda Prasad, one of the world's foremost authorities on zinc, says that the best test for deficiency is a functional one. Since one sign of deficiency is white spots on the fingernails, if your child has such spots an easy functional test would be to give your child a zinc supplement and see whether the spots disappear

Jon was a seven-year-old boy with a history of bed-wetting, colds, and behavioural problems. He didn't sleep well, his attention span was poor and he was hyperactive. He also had dry skin and his fingernails were marked with white spots. His parents were giving him cod-liver oil and vitamin C, with no observable improvement.

When I measured the level of vitamin A in Jon's blood, I found that, despite the cod-liver oil, it was low. Because the body needs zinc to use vitamin A, and because of the white spots on his nails, I suspected that Jon was zinc deficient. I used a new, very accurate and non-traumatic test of zinc status: a measurement of zinc in sweat. It confirmed the deficiency. Since Jon couldn't swallow pills, I recommended 10-mg zinc lozenges. Jon sucked on one lozenge a day, and over the next two months, he developed fewer colds and fewer white spots and his skin became less dry. His blood vitamin A levels increased to normal.

Recommended forms. Because excessive zinc supplementation lowers the body's level of such other key minerals as iron, copper, selenium and manganese, and because high zinc levels can also elevate cholesterol, I don't recommend zinc supplementation lightly. When it does seem necessary, I recommend that zinc be taken as part of a multi-mineral preparation.

Zinc lozenges are effective when a child can't swallow pills, but she should take the companion minerals listed below. Zinc lozenges also have a local anti-viral effect and are useful in treating viral (non-strep) sore throats. A child can suck on up to six a day for three or four days.

Unless your child is under supervision by a doctor with a knowledge of nutrition, *her daily dose should not be more than 10 mg*. If white spots on her nails persist after two months of this supplement, she either needs a higher dose or her nail problem is caused by something other than zinc deficiency. If she needs a higher dose, this should only be given under a doctor's supervision.

Minerals that go with zinc. To prevent depletion of other minerals because of zinc supplementation, your child's multi-mineral supplement should also include:

copper	1 mg
manganese	10 mg (manganese is poorly absorbed from supplements after the first six months of life)
selenium	75 μg (micrograms)
chromium	200 μg
molybdenum	200 μg

Chromium protects against heart disease, diabetes, and hypoglycaemia. Chromium supplements have normalized the blood sugar of diabetics and hypoglycaemics. Molybdenum helps the body use of sulphur, a substance found in all tissue, which is critical to normal immune function and to anti-oxidant activity.

Many people seem to be 'allergic' to sulphites, which are added to many foods and drinks (including squashes, wines and lettuce) as preservatives. Dr Carl Pfeiffer, of the Brain-Bio Center, Princeton, New Jersey, has found that such people usually have a molybdenum deficiency and are thus unable to break down sulphites properly. Instead of an allergy, they have a metabolism problem.

Chromium is found in whole grains and in brewer's yeast; molybdenum in meats, whole grains, pulses and leafy vegetables.

Iodine

Although essential for normal thyroid functioning, excess amounts of iodine can cause acne and contribute to the development of a thyroid inflammation called thyroiditis. If your child eats seafood, she won't need iodine or kelp supplements. If she doesn't eat seafood, a pinch of powdered kelp or 60 micrograms (μg) of iodine daily in a multivitamin will be enough.

Iron

Also a key mineral, it is crucial both to brain functioning and in maintaining a high volume of red blood cells to carry oxygen to the body's tissues. In addition to anaemia, with its attendant listlessness, iron deficiency can affect a child's capacity to think and remember, and so affect her school performance.

A good screening test for iron deficiency is a check by a doctor on the level of ferritin – the protein that stores iron – in the blood. Children with low ferritin levels, while they may not be anaemic, tend not to function well intellectually compared to children with normal levels.[2]

Alice, age six, was not exactly in wonderland when I saw her. She was tired all the time, and far behind the other children in school. When I investigated her eating habits, I discovered that she drank about 2½ pints (1.3 l) of milk a day, in addition to yoghurt, cheese and ice cream. She was borderline anaemic with a very low blood ferritin level, and her red blood cells were somewhat small and pale.

I advised her parents to cut down on the dairy products that Alice ate and drank so that she would be hungry enough for other foods. Ice cream and cheese were the first to go since they had the least to offer. Milk and yoghurt were restricted to between-meal snacks.

In addition to remedying Alice's iron deficiency, I wanted to change her eating habits so the problem wouldn't crop up again. But she didn't like the taste of meat and she didn't like to chew. I advised her parents that they prepare soft, flavourful stews with bits of meat or clams or oysters.

I also suggested a teaspoon (5 ml) of blackstrap (cane) molasses in Alice's breakfast cereal to provide iron and calcium. But blackstrap molasses is an acquired taste, and Alice wouldn't acquire it. So I prescribed a chewable multivitamin with iron, plus a chewable vitamin C – both twice a day with meals for maximum absorption. Within a month, Alice was like a new girl.

Iron is best obtained from foods, in combination with other minerals. Meat, poultry and shellfish are the best sources. Eggs contain some iron, but not in a form readily available to the body. Vitamin C increases iron absorption, so it's a good idea to serve vitamin C-rich fruits and vegetables with eggs, meat and iron-fortified cereal.

TO GET 15 MG OF IRON A DAY FROM FOOD:

Serve 2 portions from this list (3 mg of iron each)

Tuna	10 oz (275 mg)
Turkey, dark	4 oz (115 g)
Red meat	4 oz (115 g)
Pumpkin seeds	2½ tbsp (30 g)
Almonds	2¾ oz (80 g)
Sunflower seeds	2¾ oz (80 g)
Soya or kidney beans	5½ oz (160 g)
Spinach	3 oz (85 g)
Peas	8 oz (225 g)
Tomato juice	8 fl. oz (230 ml)

Serve 3 portions from this list (about 1 mg of iron each)

Egg	1
Chicken	4 oz (115 g)
Salmon, tinned	2½ oz (70 g)
Porridge	
Wholewheat muffin	1
Shredded wheat biscuit	1
Brown rice	
Tofu	2 oz (55 g)
Lentils	
Broccoli	3 oz (85 g)
Potato (medium)	1
Peanuts	2 oz (55 g)
Brazil nuts	1 oz (30 g)
Hazel nuts	3 oz (85 g)

Iron Supplements. I don't recommend an iron supplement for school-age children who aren't actually iron-deficient. Unneeded iron blocks the absorption of zinc, manganese and molybdenum, undermining the immune system.

If your child is iron-deficient, the best way to deal with it is to feed her foods rich in iron: red meat three or more times a week for a month, chilli con carne (beans with ground or chopped meat) often. Give her tomatoes, broccoli or citrus fruits with meat so that the vitamin C can increase the amount of iron she absorbs.

Or you can use a supplement. Your child should have about 15 mg of iron a day. It's best to give an iron supplement with food, but not with bran, which prevents absorption. Unless she eats a high-bran cereal for breakfast, give her iron at breakfast and supper. After three months, have her ferritin level tested again.

FIGHTING THE JUNK-FOOD JUNKIES

Junk food is ubiquitous in our culture, and sooner or later your child is going to want to eat it. She'll be exposed to it on TV, at the supermarket, at friends' houses – even, sadly, at school. Increasingly, she'll be spending most of her days away from home, and will have to deal with the temptations of junk food on her own. What can you do? Plenty.

• Don't bring junk food into the house. If your child asks for it, explain carefully and patiently that you love her and for that reason will only bring healthy food into the house.

• Limit her TV viewing to a few hours on weekends. Television advertising is particularly difficult for a child to resist because it conveys seductive images and a lot of subliminal messages. You can explain to her that TV adverts exaggerate because they are designed to sell what they're advertising.

• Provide lots of colourful, chewy, healthy snacks such as carrot sticks, courgettes, cucumber, cherry tomatoes, cauliflower and broccoli florets, and green and red pepper chunks with yoghurt or nut butter dip, oatmeal biscuits, popcorn sprinkled with grated cheese, chickpeas, wholewheat muffins, mini-pizzas, tortillas and tacos, low-fat yoghurt with fresh fruit, smoothies, muesli bars, fruit-and-nut balls, and fruit ice lollies (*see* Chapter 10). Your child and her friends can help make many of these snacks, which is half the fun.

• Eat a healthy diet yourself. Your example can work for or against you. If you tell your child not to eat what you eat, she's going to wonder about the double standards. And she's not going to believe you if you tell her that adults are immune from the harmful effects of bad food. If you snack on crisps, she's not going to see anything wrong with them no matter what you tell her.

• If you're eating the same kind of healthy diet that you expect her to eat, start explaining what's behind it. Tell her a healthy body needs protein, vitamins, minerals and the right oils for peak performance, and that these things come from vegetables, fruits, whole grains, seafood, poultry and so forth – not from sugar and fat. She can understand that sugar and fat just fill her up without giving her body any of the nutrients it needs. Stress the importance of good food for the attributes that are important to her: Good food will make her feel good and look good. It will help her to be smart and strong and athletic, and will help keep her from getting sick.

• Assert your rights at school: visit the school to find out what your child is being encouraged to eat there. Visit the lunchroom during lunch hour. If the situation is not what you would want, have a frank talk with your child's teacher and the head teacher. Join the PTA or other parents' group and campaign for healthier school dinners. (In addition, as we discussed on pp. 124–126, you could send your child to school with a packed lunch.)

• To help her cope with the different eating patterns of other families, tell her that, while other families have other ideas about what to eat, you expect the parents of other children to respect your ideas about what is best for your children. A child who believes that you love her and want her to eat right so that she can become strong and successful in school will be more likely to follow your guidance even when you're out of sight. You're still the major authority figure in her life, so when she's with friends whose parents may offer foods that you would not allow her to have, she'll be able to say 'No, thank you' easily and courteously because she wants to please you.

• Discuss nutrition with the parents of your child's friends and with your child's care giver (e.g. her childminder) if any. You may find that, while many of them agree with you in principle, they feel they have no control over their children much of the time, or just give in to social pressure. Explain your position to them and seek some common ground. Obviously, if your child eats meals at another house, you expect her to eat what she's served. Explain your thoughts about the worst anti-nutrients: fizzy drinks, crisps, sweets and sweet junk foods. Request that these items not be offered to your child.

If your child is well-fed by you all week, a weekend party at which she's fed Coke, gooey cake and ice cream by someone else's parents won't harm her. Good friends are as important as good food, maybe more so. Explain to your child that, by eating well all week, she is, in fact, being fortified against the effects of weekend indulgence at those parties that mean so much to her.

USING NUTRITION TO COPE WITH SPECIAL PROBLEMS

OBESITY

My basic diet plan doesn't provide the empty calories that can lead to obesity, but you may have a problem if your child is very inactive, if she craves sweets and eats junk food away from home, or – an unlikely occurrence – if she eats too much of the healthy food you serve her. Since obesity is a major problem among school-age children today, how can you nip the problem in the bud? You need a dual approach: through activity and through food.

You also need to realize that children want to be like their parents, so you *must* set a good example. It's crucial that you eat the same kinds of healthy foods that you expect your child to eat. Stress how important it is to be healthy and to grow up strong and resistant to illness. If you are changing your eating habits, let your child know how much better you feel. Take the lead in physical activity and include her and the rest of the family. You may have to change your own lifestyle, but it will be well worth it.

At seven, Mack was a bit chubby and a poor eater. He was a sedentary child who liked very few foods. At school, he would trade his packed lunch for biscuits and sweets. In fact, he wasn't much different from his mother.

I realized that there wasn't any point in trying to change Mack's behaviour; this was a family problem. I enlisted his mother in the project. She had to confront her own style of eating and her own sedentary habits, but as she began to make changes, she enlisted Mack as a 'buddy'. They exercised together and began to plan healthy menus together. Mack started helping with the cooking.

Within a few months, the family's habits were very different, and Mack was a changed child. He began to feel good about himself, not only because he looked and felt better but also because he was not the object of a prescription for change. He was an agent in a positive family process.

Activity

Some children are born more active than others. If your child is relatively inactive by nature, you can help by creating opportunities for physical activity, by being active yourself, and by helping your child find some area of movement that pleases her. She may be able to choose swimming, netball, hockey, rounders, or other games. If they are available where you live or go on holiday, skating and skiing are excellent forms of exercise, as is country dancing.

Sharing activity can provide motivation for both of you. The whole family can take brisk walks, cycle, go swimming, play ball games, or ski or skate together. You can follow an aerobics programme on TV with your child, or dance to music. Your child should engage in some brisk activity every day, and it won't hurt you, either.

Of course, all these suggestions are useful for active children and parents too. Sharing activities is a great way to share love and good feelings.

Be sure to praise your child for all her physical activity. This is crucial.

Food

In addition to all the tips I give above, under 'Fighting the junk-food junkies' there are some more useful tips for dealing with an overweight child.

Never force her to eat or tell her to 'clean her plate'. Don't bargain with her either, and never use sweets or dessert as a reward or treat. Saying, 'You have to finish all your food to get dessert' will just make dessert seem like the best part of the meal. In fact, encourage her to stop eating when she feels full. That way, she'll learn not to overeat. Encourage her to eat slowly by putting down her fork between bites and chewing deliberately. If she's a fast eater, this may take time to master, but the rewards are better digestion and a more relaxed meal. Do the same thing yourself.

Call foods 'healthy' and 'unhealthy' rather than 'fattening' and 'non-fattening'. Tell her that you don't eat junk foods because your body is not a rubbish dump. Praise her when she chooses healthy foods.

Encourage her to eat the lower-calorie healthy foods – fish, poultry, potatoes, vegetables and fresh fruit – rather than the higher-calorie items such as nuts, seeds, dried fruits, fruit juices, cheese and milk.

Don't display tempting items such as biscuits, nuts or crisps in your home. Don't keep a glass biscuit jar out on an open shelf, for instance. Don't keep sweets at all.

If your child craves sugary or salty foods, encourage her to notice the varied tastes of the well-prepared foods you serve. Sweet and salt are not necessarily acquired tastes, but eating lots of sweet or salty foods numbs the palate to more delicate and subtle flavours. The less she eats sweets, the less she will crave them. Gradually, the nutritious, naturally sweet desserts you learn to make will come to seem sweet enough to satisfy her – and you.

Above all, *don't* encourage dieting. Weight depends on overall eating patterns and levels of activity – and crash diets can be harmful. Anorexia and bulimia (self-starvation and binge eating followed by vomiting) are major problems among adolescent girls (and some boys) today, and the eating habits and skewed self-images that lead to these problems are being formed in childhood.

Overweight children tend to have very poor self-images. If your child is overweight, one of the most important things you can do is to help her develop a better self-image. *Never* call attention to her weight; instead, talk to her about how she feels about herself. Point out her positive traits: is she funny, friendly, cooperative, caring, sharing, affectionate, inventive, loyal, a good student, a good listener, musical, clever, good with her hands, fun to take on trips and share adventures with, athletic, artistic?

Like Mack, all children feel better if they are involved in the nutritional changes made by their parents. Discuss the nutritional value of foods with your child so she can help you plan menus. Get her involved in preparing food, too.

ALLERGIES

If your child has chronically itchy skin, eyes, or anus, frequent skin rashes or dark circles under her eyes, she may have an allergy. Snoring and nasal congestion that seem to be a reaction to cats, dogs, plants or such indoor spaces as cellars or barns are also symptoms. So are abdominal pains, headaches, chronic fatigue, asthma and some behavioural problems.

Allergies are helped by my basic diet, including linseed oil and a magnesium supplement. In young children, headaches and abdominal pain particularly suggest a magnesium deficiency. I would give them 3 mg per pound of body weight every day as a supplement. If that doesn't work, double the dose.

Allergic children often become less allergic if they supplement their diets with the co-factor nutrients required for proper EFA metabolism and with anti-oxidants to decrease allergic inflammation:

vitamin A	5000 mg daily (as beta-carotene)
vitamin B_6	10 mg daily
vitamin E	100 units daily
vitamin C	500 mg daily
zinc	10 mg daily
copper	1 mg daily
manganese	10 mg daily
selenium	75 µg daily

Food

To detect a food allergy, follow these steps, focusing on two specific items:

• *Milk.* As the most common food allergen, this is the place to start. If your child drinks a lot of milk or eats a lot of cheese or yoghurt, try the five-day elimination diet. Eliminate from your child's diet *all* milk, butter, cream, cheese, yoghurt, ice cream and any foods containing milk, milk solids or milk derivatives. Read all labels carefully to look for whey or sodium caseinate, derived from the milk protein casein. (For more on milk-elimination diets, *see* p. 69–70.)

• *Yeast.* If your child begins to show *some* improvement on the five-day milk-elimination diet, stay with it and begin to investigate yeast. If there is no improvement, drop the milk-free diet and check out yeast. A child who has had antibiotics more than once a year, who has *any type* of allergy, who has behavioural problems of any kind, or who develops behavioural problems *after* antibiotic treatment might have a yeast sensitization problem.

As I explained in Chapter 6, antibiotics destroy the good intestinal bacteria that normally kill yeast. When a child becomes sensitive or allergic to this yeast overgrowth (*Candida albicans* is the species of yeast involved), the sensitivity can extend to other types of yeast and to moulds, and can intensify *any* allergic problems, from asthma to hyperactivity. A yeast-elimination diet can help identify the culprit.

It's important to limit natural sugar, including dried fruits and commercial fruit juices. Sugar aggravates a yeast allergy by stimulating yeast growth in the mouth. (As you will see next, dried fruits and commercial fruit juices are full of yeast, too, so you will want to eliminate them.)

To check for an allergy to the yeast and mould found in food, you will have to eliminate many other items from your child's diet. Yeast and mould are found in most cheeses, breads and biscuits; they are also used as additives in pasta, bread and many canned items (including soups, which may contain yeast extract); eliminate these.

Yeast grows naturally on the skins of such fruits and vegetables as peaches, apples and tomatoes. So products made from them, such as fruit juices, dried fruits and tomato sauce are all pretty yeasty. Peel fresh fruits and vegetables, and prepare fresh orange or grapefruit juice yourself. Eliminate canned or bottled fruit juices if you haven't already, and fruits (such as berries) that can't be peeled.

Vinegar is made by the action of yeast, and it can be found in pickles, ketchup, mustard, mayonnaise, barbecue sauces and salad dressings. Eliminate all of them.

Vitamins may also contain yeast; make sure your child's are yeast-free.

Malt, another yeast product, is used as a flavouring in many breakfast cereals. Restrict your child to oatmeal, puffed wheat and puffed rice. Read labels of drinks to be sure malt hasn't been used as a flavouring.

Your child *can* eat meat, poultry, fish, eggs, rice, oats, peeled fresh vegetables and fruit (limit fresh fruit to two pieces a day), and such yeast-free grain products as cream crackers.

Keep your child on this diet of 'safe foods' for five days. Then re-introduce, one at a time, vinegary foods, dried fruit, bread, commercial fruit juices and cheese for two days. If your child improves during the five-day elimination and deteriorates when yeasty foods are re-introduced, she may have an allergy to yeast in food.

If the elimination diet helps, keep it up for a while. If it doesn't, or causes too much resistance, you have two choices:

● Consult a doctor who works with food allergy. The organization Action Against Allergy (43 The Downs, London SW20 8HG, tel: 01-947 5082) should be able to help.

● If your child has had lots of antibiotics or you've seen allergies develop or get worse after antibiotics, you can take steps to decrease intestinal yeast growth nutritionally.

On your own, you can restrict artificial and natural sugar: no honey, dried fruit, fruit juice, sugar-loaded drinks, cakes, etc., and no more than two pieces of fruit a day. *Acidophilus*, a bacteria normally found in the large intestine, helps keep down yeast growth there; you can buy supplements of this at healthfood shops.

Asthma

This is one of the most difficult problems that commonly afflict young children; at worst, its effects can be tragic – a crippling loss of breath, even death. Fortunately though, most of the time it can be treated with nutrition and without drugs. If an effective allergy-desensitization technique is used, and as much environmental control as possible is exercised, drug-free treatment is virtually always possible in children.

Here are some guidelines for asthma treatment:

• Put your child on my basic low-sugar healthy diet.
• Linseed oil: 1 tablespoon (15 ml) daily
• Magnesium: 3 mg per pound of body weight each day
• Eliminate milk and all milk products and derivatives. (Many asthmatics are allergic to milk.) Give a 600-mg calcium supplement each day.
• If there is a history of antibiotics or hydrocortisone use (there usually is), check for a yeast problem and treat it as described above, pp. 141–142
• The following nutritional supplements have been found to play a definite role in asthma:

—*Fatty acids:* High doses of fish oils suppress the formation of leukotrienes, which cause the bronchial tubes to constrict. I recommend 1 tablespoon (15 ml) of cod-liver oil or, better yet, 3 grams of MaxEPA (fish-oil-extract capsules) a day.

—*High doses of vitamin C:* About 2 grams a day help to improve the flow of air by dilating the bronchial tubes through an indirect effect on prostaglandin formation; a reduction in histamine levels also occurs.[3]

—*Vitamin B_6:* A study at the world-famous Cleveland Clinic showed that asthmatic patients have difficulty maintaining vitamin B_6 (pyridoxine) in its active form. A dose of 200 mg a day helps these patients.[4]

—*Vitamin B_{12}:* Low levels of vitamin B_{12} have been found in studies of asthmatic children who lacked stomach acid. High doses of B_{12} given by daily injection have cured some of the more severe and unresponsive asthmatics, with the best results occurring in children. The dose is 1 mg twice a day for about six weeks (*ouch!*). Fortunately, I have not had to use this method since others often work so well.

COMMON INFECTIONS

Health isn't the absence of disease; it's the ability to overcome it. As they grow up, healthy children catch and get over a number of infections. Because of immunization, many childhood diseases have virtually disappeared, but colds and flu are still common. These are viral infections, and they need no specific treatment. In fact, the worst thing to do is to treat a viral infection with antibiotics – these drugs have absolutely no effect on the virus and they just encourage yeast infections. Aspirin may help lower fever and relieve pain, but it increases the length of viral infections. Fever is actually a protective mechanism, and I would not lower a child's temperature unless it goes over 103° F (39.4° C) or the child is in a lot of pain. (At this age, febrile convulsions are rare.)

At ten, Sam had a continually stuffy nose and complained about frequent stomach aches and headaches. He said he felt 'sick' most of the time. His parents had found that food made him sick, and had put him on a very limited diet that avoided most fruits, dairy products, cereals and eggs. Despite this diet, though, he still felt ill most days.

Right after coming to see me, Sam caught flu. I recommended that his parents not give him aspirin or paracetamol to suppress his fever, and they let it run its course over several days. When it was over, Sam was completely well – he had no symptoms of allergy at all. He remained in 'remission' for six months.

You can diminish the severity of colds and flu with vitamins C and A in higher-than-nutritional doses: 1000 to 2000 mg (1 to 2 grams) of vitamin C a day; 10,000 international units of vitamin A. These doses can safely be given for two weeks.

The truth is that healthy children benefit from occasional virus infections, and should be allowed to experience them. The exception is a child who has chronic or recurrent colds, frequent sore throats (caused by either bacteria or viruses) or asthma. In such children, viral infections further weaken the immune system instead of strengthening it. What they need are immune boosters.

Immune boosters

If your child catches everything that comes around, I recommend the following in addition to my basic meal plan, linseed oil and magnesium:

● **Vitamin C.** When your child gets a virus, the vitamin C levels in her body drop. School-age children (5–10 years old) can safely take up to 2000 mg (2 grams) a day. After that, let your child's body fight the virus. When she gets better, taper the vitamin C back down to 500 mg a day. Doses of vitamin C in the 1000- to 3000-mg-a-day range enhance immune function in healthy people.[5]

● **Vitamin A.** Carotene, the form of vitamin A found in plants, is an effective anti-oxidant. Retinol, the form of vitamin A in animal foods, supports the action of your child's killer T-cells. Virus infections deplete a child's vitamin

A stores.[6] Administer 10,000 international units a day in a capsule, or 1 teaspoon (5 ml) of cod-liver oil a day, or increase her intake of vitamin A from animal sources (liver, eggs, butter), using the guidelines on page 89.

• **Zinc and iron.** The importance of these minerals for immune function was explained on pages 84–87. Increase the amount of zinc and iron your child gets in food, using the guidelines on pages 85–86, or supplement her diet with the minerals as described on page 87.

• **Fish oils.** If your child has more than two respiratory infections a year and her skin is dry despite linseed oil, she may not be able to use linseed oil well as a source of omega-3 EFAs. Try using fish oils. A teaspoon (5 ml) of old-fashioned Norwegian cod-liver oil for a five-year-old to a tablespoon (15 ml) for a 12-year-old will serve and will supply plenty of vitamins A and D as well – so cut out the liver supplements.

Alternatively, you can give her fish-oil capsules (e.g. MaxEPA), 2 to 3 grams per day. The omega-3s in fish oils are chemically different from those in linseed oil. They are more unsaturated – in fact, they're the most natural unsaturated oils that exist. Some children, especially those with allergies, cannot form these extra-unsaturated EFAs well themselves, and need to consume fish oils to compensate.

In addition

• **Water.** When she's sick, don't force your child to eat, but make sure she drinks plenty of fluids to prevent dehydration; pure water and freshly-squeezed juice are good, or dilute concentrated fruit juice with water.

• **Yeast.** If she's had lots of antibiotics, check out a possible yeast problem. I've described the specific steps for this investigation above, under 'Allergies'.

• **Allergy.** Look for indications of an allergy: itchy skin, eyes or anus; skin rashes; dark circles under the eyes. Also snoring, and nasal congestion related to the environment (the presence of cats or dogs, being in barns or cellars, or attending parties) or the season.

HYPERACTIVITY

The most common behavioural problem that children at this age have is adjusting to school. In many cases, there may be a comparatively simple reason: often, a child is emotionally immature for the demands placed on her age level at school. This is especially likely to happen to a bright child, whose intellectual development exceeds her chronological age and whose social development lags behind both.

I believe such a child should not be pushed ahead; she may, in fact, greatly benefit from being allowed to repeat a year so that her social development can catch up to that of her peers (although I realize that this is only now being discussed as an option for British schools). If this is suggested for your child, don't let a feeling of false pride keep you from making a decision to let your child repeat a year. Some of the happiest, best-adjusted kids I know were immature in their first year at school, repeated it and have made steady, successful progress since.

Then there are the children whose problems involve irritability, short attention spans and generally difficult behaviour. These children are often called *hyperactive* or are considered to be suffering from an *attention-deficit disorder*. Until the 1970s, such children were often called bad, lazy or stupid. Now it is recognized that they need help – and, increasingly, that their problems may be biochemical in origin. Behavioural difficulties of this type can have a psychological or social background, such as the stress of a divorce. But when a troubled child's home is stable, my experience has shown that nutrition and food allergy often play important roles.

For instance, Peter couldn't sit still in class, and he constantly whistled or made popping noises. The minute he felt frustrated or was rebuked, he would burst into tears. He wet his bed every night, and he had a terrible self-image. Although he loved milk and drank about two pints a day, he was thirsty all the time. The dark circles under his eyes suggested an allergy.

I suspected Peter's problem was milk, one of the most potent food allergens in young children, so I recommended that he go for five days without milk, butter, cheese, yoghurt, ice cream or any other foods containing milk, milk solids or milk derivatives. (Milk derivatives such as commercial ice cream include whey and casein. Casein is also often added to package foods as sodium caseinate.) Instead, he got water and diluted juice.

Peter didn't like this change very much, and he was no more attentive in school. But he stopped making popping noises, and he stopped bed-wetting. These were significant changes, clues that we were on the right track towards finding the ultimate culprit. Peter actually had many allergies and the usual deficiencies of magnesium and EFAs.

To help your hyperactive child, you'll need to do a little detective work. Ask the following questions:
● Is her diet healthy, or does she eat lots of sugar and junk foods? To be a sugar sleuth, you must read the ingredients on prepared foods. Most of the

sugar eaten by kids is not table sugar; it is hidden in food by the manufacturer. The following are all fundamentally sugar: *dextrose, corn sweetener, corn syrup, fructose* and *honey*. Don't use foods that include any of these among the first five ingredients.

- Is she very thirsty?
- Does she regularly wet her bed?
- Does she have dry hair or skin?
- Has she had antibiotics recently, or has she had several antibiotic treatments in her life?
- Are there any foods, such as milk or vinegar, that she seems to crave?
- Does she have allergic symptoms such as puffy eyes, runny nose, cough, itchy skin?
- Is there a family history of allergy?

If the answer to any of these questions is *yes*, it's time to begin work. The three critical nutritional areas you will investigate are *EFAs, magnesium* and *food allergies*.

EFAs

First, eliminate junk food from your child's diet. Follow the diet plan in this chapter for a low-sugar, nutritionally rich diet supplemented with linseed oil, 1 tablespoon (15 ml) a day (or substitute 1 teaspoon/15 ml of cod-liver oil or 2 tablespoons/30 ml of walnut oil), to provide omega-3 EFAs. Get food-grade linseed oil. It should be almost tasteless; if it tastes at all bitter, it is rancid – throw it out. (*See* Chapter 1 for a full discussion of EFAs and linseed oil.)

If your child has a specific EFA deficiency, she may be excessively thirsty, her skin may be dry and her hair may be dull and lifeless. If linseed or walnut or cod-liver oil is the key to correcting her deficiency, you will know after a month: her thirst will be back to normal, her skin will be smoother, her hair silkier and more lustrous.

If, on the other hand, your child becomes *thirstier* with the linseed or walnut or cod-liver oil at any point from a few days to a month, the deficiency may involve omega-6 EFAs. Such children are usually hyperactive *boys*; they may have enzymes that are so sensitive to omega-3 EFAs that the small amount provided by the usual Western diet is actually enough for them. Stop the oil you are using and substitute safflower oil: 1 tablespoon (15 ml) a day. Or, better still, give your child evening primrose oil (two to three 500-mg capsules a day), or two to three 250-mg capsules of blackcurrant seed oil.

Be careful when you buy primrose oil; it's so expensive that bogus cut-rate brands have begun to appear. They are useless. I recommend sticking with the Efamol brand.

If primrose or blackcurrant seed oil is going to help at all for different specific problems, you should expect to see results as follows:

- Excessive thirst, restless sleep: a return to normal patterns within 72 hours.
- Bed-wetting: expect a change for the better within a week.
- Other behavioural problems will take about a month – again, *if the oil is going to help at all.*
- Dry skin and hair will take about two weeks.

Should you raise the dosage if a child shows no improvement, or improves in only one area? I'm often asked this question, and my advice is that if three 500-mg capsules of primrose oil or three 250-mg capsules of blackcurrant seed oil a day produce a beneficial change in *any* area, it means that the oil is having some effect. Therefore, *don't* raise the dosage – just give the oil more time to work. Too much of these oils has been known actually to *reverse* the beneficial effect.

But if you see absolutely no change in *any* area after three weeks, then raise the dose by one pill a day, give that dosage for seven days, then add one more pill for seven days, and continue adding one pill a week until your child is taking a *maximum* of six pills a day. If there is still no effect, go on to the next step.

Magnesium

The next step is to give your child a magnesium supplement. Give 3 mg per pound per day in the form of enteric-coated magnesium chloride tablets (this will involve the taking of two to six pills a day) or as magnesium citrate liquid – 1 to 2 tablespoons (15–30 ml) daily or capsules (one to three daily). Do this *in addition to* the primrose or linseed oil; the two may have an additive effect.

Calcium

If your child drinks *less* than 16 fluid ounces (460 ml) of milk a day, or eats less than its equivalent in yoghurt, add a calcium supplement according to the instructions on p. 83.

Not recommended. Megavitamin therapy is usually not at all helpful with hyperactive children; in fact, it often makes their behaviour worse. The B-vitamins are especially tricky: some children are allergic to the yeast used in making most B-complex tablets or capsules; others simply have adverse reactions to the B-vitamins themselves. I've found that hyperactive children are generally also hypersensitive; they overract to stimuli, whether chemical, sensory or emotional. In fact, they are living examples of the unity of mind and body. Instead of pouring more supplements into their bodies, now is the time to do some allergy detective work.

Food allergies

It is well-established that allergies to foods and food additives, and to inhaled chemicals and mould spores, play a role in hyperactivity. (For a fuller discussion of the scientific evidence for this, *see* Chapter 6, pp. 111–117.) Once you've tested for the effects of EFAs and added magnesium to your child's diet, some food trials are in order. (Follow the procedure outlined on pp. 69–70.)

Jethro was a child whose behavioural problems stemmed entirely from a yeast overgrowth as a result of antibiotics. At eight, he wasn't a bad-natured child, but his frenetic behaviour drove his mother crazy. He had been a normal baby until he had a couple of ear infections. Both responded to antibiotics, but after the second one, and two courses of antibiotics, Jethro at 18 months became a changed child. Instead of the bright, alert boy he had been, he became inattentive during the day and restless and wakeful at night. For a while, his parents thought he would outgrow this behaviour; instead, it became worse. Jethro began to wet his bed. He had a hard time getting to sleep and was hard to get up in the morning. He seemed intolerant of changes and had problems adjusting to school. Because of his poor record, he was being evaluated for a special-education programme.

We laid out a strategy that included:
- a balanced low-sugar diet
- an acidophilus supplement

During the first four to six weeks of this treatment, Jethro's behaviour gradually improved. His school performance went from consistently poor to variable – he now had good days as well as bad ones, and the bad ones weren't as bad as they had been.

At this point, we put Jethro on the yeast and mould elimination diet, and it worked wonders. In fact, he became a new child – or, perhaps, just the child he had been becoming before he was sidetracked by his ear infections and antibiotics.

The earlier you treat problems such as hyperactivity or asthma with sound nutrition, the better the results of the treatment will be and the more cooperation you are likely to get from your child. Adolescents are particularly wilful and rebellious – their special needs are described in the next chapter.

Ages 13 to 17:
Keeping Your Teenager
in Top Health

Adolescence is hard on parents and adolescents alike. You've been feeding your child a healthy diet and he has been getting plenty of exercise. But now he may skip lunch at school to hang out with the other kids at the local fish-and-chip shop. He's not interested in vegetables: given a choice, he'll go for anything sweet and sugary or fried and fatty. He is *certainly* not willing to go to school with a nutritious sandwich in a packed lunch. Unless he goes out for school sports, he's probably not getting a lot of exercise, either. He'll do anything to cadge a lift rather than walk or ride his bike.

Throughout his adolescence, he'll have to make difficult choices concerning cigarettes, alcohol, drugs, sex and ethics (whether or not he should be honest about doing homework or in dealing with other people, both his peers and adults, including you). He wants very much to believe in your values, but at his age, example is more crucial than ever. If you skip breakfast, why shouldn't he? If you can't take the time for regular exercise, why should he? If you have a drink to relax at the end of the day, why shouldn't he? You can, of course, forbid him to drink and exhort him to exercise, but in the absence of your positive example, he's bound to discount your words. What's more, you'll be undermining one of the most precious things in your relationship: his belief in you.

Your teenager's self-interest provides you with a couple of points in favour of good nutrition: He's starting to care a great deal about his looks. He's worried about his skin, his hair and his physique. The best road to a lean body, clear skin, lustrous hair and shining eyes is, of course, through nutrition and exercise. If your teenager is an athlete, a little clear information should help convince him that good nutrition is essential for top-notch performance. In fact, a teenager is well able to absorb the basic nutritional information in the first chapter of this book, and in this chapter as well.

Your teenager is under a lot of pressure: His hormones are creating immense physiological changes to which he must adjust while also heeding pressure to succeed academically, socially and perhaps athletically. Peer pressures are especially intense at this age, and the choices he faces are more than difficult; they have potentially dangerous consequences, from addiction to AIDS. In the pages that follow, I will offer guidelines to help you cope with one important area that affects what happens to him in all the other aspects of his life: nutrition. If he is getting the best nutrition you can give him, he will be in a better position to cope with the stresses of the rest of his life. All his systems, including his immune system, will be 'go'.

It should go without saying that your teenager needs lots of love and attention. He may not always be able to ask for it, so sharpen your sensitivity and learn to be there before you are called.

THE SPECIAL NUTRITIONAL NEEDS OF ADOLESCENTS

A teenager's tendency to forget such things as fresh vegetables exist makes the usual teen diet much too low in folic acid, vitamin A and essential fatty acids – all crucial to the health of his immune system. What's more, sexual development in boys increases their need for zinc, which is concentrated in semen. The zinc that is lost in ejaculation must be replaced through nutrition. Rising levels of oestrogen in girls produce changes in the way their bodies handle vitamin B_6 and magnesium. As a result, they need more of both.

But if your teenage son or daughter is eating a lot of lunches and snacks with the group at McDonald's, what are you going to do? Well, first of all, it's not the end of the world. It would be worse if he or she didn't have any friends. Concentrate on the meals you can control – breakfast, dinner and (sometimes) afterschool snacks. And give him some basic supplements. Although I don't advocate a broad programme of preventive nutritional supplementation for younger children, I do think it is worthwhile for adolescents.

DIETARY ESSENTIALS FOR YOUR ADOLESCENT

Your teenager needs a moderate amount of protein, a lot of fibre and minerals, and very little fat, sugar and salt. Many studies in the last few years have linked fats to cancer, heart disease, high blood pressure (hypertension), arthritis and multiple sclerosis. Marbled red meats and pork and such high-fat dairy products as whole milk and cheese should be served seldom and in small amounts.

A diet high in salt may contribute to hypertension and strokes. Sugar supplies calories without nutrients and contributes to obesity as well as to several vitamin and mineral deficiencies.

THE TRUTH ABOUT CALCIUM AND STRONG BONES: *or Why a Pepsi or Coke is the worst thing for your teenage daughter*

Osteoporosis is a major health problem among women. Most begin losing bone density at menopause, but whether or not they actually develop osteoporosis depends to a great extent on how dense their bones are before that. A woman has about 20 years to develop dense bones – from puberty to her early 30s. After the age of 35, it's too late to build bone density; she can only try to prevent bone loss.

Two factors help build dense bones in adolescence: *exercise* and *diet*. Weight-bearing activities such as walking, running or playing tennis, which put pressure on bones, especially the legs and spine, stimulate the formation of new bone tissue. Swimming, which puts no pressure on bones, does not help prevent osteoporosis.

Walking is an excellent exercise, available to everybody. I encourage regular family walks – at least a half an hour a day. It's a good way to spend time with your kids and a healthy habit.

Nutrition for building healthy bones starts with calcium, the major bone mineral. But calcium alone is not enough; the right amounts of several key co-factor nutrients are needed: protein, phosphorus, magnesium, manganese, copper, silica and vitamins A and D.

The first step in forming new bone is the laying down of a soft, rubbery protein called *bone matrix*. Crystals of calcium, phosphorus and magnesium, deposited on the matrix, make it hard and rigid. The rate at which calcium is deposited depends on many nutritional and hormonal factors, the most important of which is the level of calcium in the blood. This in turn depends partly on the amount of calcium absorbed from the intestine, and *that* reflects both the amount of calcium in the diet and the amount of vitamin D in the body.

Because osteoporosis is such a big problem, women are often advised to take a lot of calcium and vitamin D. Alas, this advice is quite irrational. To understand why, we have to understand the intricate mechanisms that control the absorption and use of calcium in the body.

The level of calcium in your teenager's blood is tightly controlled by a hormone called *parathyroid hormone* (PTH), which is produced by the four tiny parathyroid glands that sit on the thyroid gland. Among other things, PTH activates vitamin D. Vitamin D is different from all other vitamins. In fact, it isn't really a vitamin at all: it's a hormone produced by the skin when it is exposed to sunlight. And to be of any use, it must be activated by PTH. Active vitamin D, or *calcitriol*, increases the rate at which calcium is absorbed from food in the intestine.

When the level of calcium in the blood falls, the parathyroid glands secrete more PTH, which in turn converts more vitamin D into calcitriol. The calcitriol increases the amount of calcium that's absorbed from food.

When the level of calcium in the blood goes up, the parathyroid glands stop secreting PTH, and the body stops making calcitriol for a while. If a person eats a lot of calcium or starts taking calcium supplements, blood calcium goes up, so PTH secretion drops and calcitriol levels fall. The result is that *less* calcium is absorbed even though there is more available in the intestines!

So if you consume only a moderate amount of calcium rather than a megadose, you'll absorb a higher percentage of it. Howard Rasmussen of Yale University, one of the world's leading calcium experts, points out that the chief effect of increasing calcium intake from 650 mg a day (the UK RDA, considered low in the United States) to 1200 mg a day (the US RDA for teenagers) is that calcitriol production falls, and so, therefore, does the percentage of calcium absorbed from the intestine. The extra calcium just goes out in the stool. (This does *not* hold true, though, for a diet that is seriously *deficient* in calcium: *650 mg a day are essential.*)

THE CRUCIAL CALCIUM CO-FACTOR NUTRIENTS

Rasmussen's observations are only valid if the calcium–PTH–calcitriol regulatory mechanism is working. It generally works less well in the elderly, but in adolescents it should work very well *if* their diets are also rich in the calcium co-factor nutrients: magnesium, phosphorus, vitamin A and essential fatty acids (EFAs).

• *Magnesium.* Magnesium is essential for the release and activity of PTH; both are impaired by magnesium deficiency.
• *Phosphorus.* A two-edged sword, it is essential for laying down bone but, in excess blocks both the secretion of PTH by the parathyroids and the absorption of calcium and magnesium from the intestines. The Western diet

is marginally low in magnesium and excessively high in phosphorus. Phosphorus is found in rich supply in meat and in preservatives. Most important for adolescents, it is used to keep nearly all soft drinks bubbly. There is nothing worse for the bones of a teenage girl than Coke or Pepsi.

● *Vitamin A and EFAs.* Both are required to enable calcitriol to do its important work in the intestinal tract.

● *Magnesium, copper and manganese* help move calcium from the blood into the bones. Unfortunately, teenagers' diets are often deficient in these minerals.

Some food sources of calcium co-factor minerals

Food sources of these important bone minerals are our old friends: seafood, beans and other pulses, vegetables, whole grains, nuts and seeds. Silica is mostly found in water; the nutritional herb horsetail (*Equisetum*) is also a rich source. Horsetail tea would be a great substitute for soft drinks. If a teaspoon of honey were needed for a teenager to accept it, the trade-off would be worth it. Other foods for healthy bones include:

FOOD	MAGNESIUM (mg)	COPPER (mg)	MANGANESE (mg)
Cod, mackerel, 4 oz (115 g)	30	1.5	trace
Brown rice, 6 oz (170 g)	45	trace	3.2
Oatmeal, 2½ oz (70 g)	75	trace	1.5
Brazil nuts, 2¼ oz (65 g)	175	1.0	2.0
Almonds, 2¼ oz (65 g)	140	0.4	1.3
Sesame seeds, 2 oz (30 g)	104	0.9	0.6
Walnuts, 2¼ oz (65 g)	95	0.5	0.7
Tofu, 4 oz (115 g)	112	0.8	1.0
Spinach, cooked 8 oz (225 g),	100	0.3	1.4

A MEAL PLAN FOR ADOLESCENTS

Your teenager needs a variety of nutritious foods: fish, poultry, lean meat, eggs, low-fat milk products, fresh and dried fruits, nuts, seeds, beans, vegetables, all types of grains (rice, maize, oats, wheat and so on).

At home, you will want to avoid serving some foods altogether:

● *Fatty foods.* Fat contains over twice as many calories per gram as carbohydrate or protein, and when it is used for frying, as for potato crisps, it is usually loaded with toxic breakdown products. In addition, most high-fat foods contain the kinds of fat that interfere with the body's ability to absorb calcium and magnesium and to metabolize EFAs. You will want to eliminate fried foods completely, also bacon, sausages, luncheon meats, commercial pizza, hard cheeses, virtually every variety of commercial crisps, cream, ice cream and margarine.

● *Sugar.* High-sugar foods include many breakfast cereals, commercial baked goods, all sweets, ketchup. Read the label on every container or package of manufactured food. If sugar, corn syrup, dextrose or fructose is one of the first few ingredients, don't buy it. And since most manufactured foods are high in salt as well as sugar, you'll kill two birds with one stone.

● *Phosphates.* Preservatives and soft drinks are high in added phosphates. Limit beef to twice a week, tops.

Here's a food plan that will enable you to feed your teenager nutritious, interesting and convenient breakfasts, after-school snacks and dinners.

BREAKFASTS

Citrus juice or cut-up orange slices – plus any of the following:
● *Cereal.* For a sweet, crunchy, high-fibre, mineral-rich and easy-to-cook cereal, mix equal parts of rolled oats and oat bran, and add small amounts of chopped walnuts, sesame and sunflower seeds, raisins and/or chopped dates. Add milk or yoghurt if desired.
● *Homemade muesli or Swiss Muesli (see Chapter 10).*
● *Nutritious sesame waffles (see Chapter 10).*
● *Blueberry wholewheat pancakes (see Chapter 10).*
● *Toasted low-sugar bran muffins (see Chapter 10).* Serve with a non-sugar fruit spread or almond butter or low-fat cottage cheese and chopped fruit.
● *Poached or boiled egg* and whole-grain toast. With the recent salmonella scare in mind, be sure to cook the eggs for at least 8 minutes.

PACKED LUNCHES FOR SCHOOL

If you can persuade your teenager to take a packed lunch, I suggest you follow the suggestions in the previous chapter, including my recommendations for types of bread.

AFTER-SCHOOL SNACKS

- *Pancakes and waffles.* Keep these in the freezer. Heat and serve with applesauce or fruit purée. If you need to use tinned fruit on occasion, be sure to buy the varieties canned in their own or another fruit's juice, or rinse off the syrup.
- *Pita bread pizza.* Fill a wholewheat pita pocket with low-fat mozzarella and fresh vegetables. Bake for five to ten minutes.
- *Unsalted mixed nuts.*
- *Mexican bean dip* served with carrot or celery sticks (*see* Chapter 10) or crisp bread. Cook in batches, freeze and thaw as needed. Do *not* use commercial crisps, which are high in fat.
- *High-protein muesli bars* (*see* Chapter 10).
- *Soup.* You can make it for immediate consumption or freeze batches for later use. Serve with whole-grain toast, crisp bread or bran muffin. Good choices for batch cooking: bean, lentil, creamy tomato.

DINNERS

Dinner is usually too large a meal and too full of protein these days. I favour lighter, low-protein suppers – one dish plus bread and salad. You can use the dinners in Chapter 7; if you have more than one child, you will want to prepare the same for both. But teenagers are sometimes willing to be more adventurous than younger children; try the following on yours. *See* recipes in Chapter 10 for seafood ratatouille, stir-fried vegetables and tofu, lentil and barley stew, or tofu-ricotta Lasagne.

DESSERTS

Check the recipe section in Chapter 10 for nutritious, low-sugar desserts. Fresh fruit is always good.

PARTIES

If you serve nutritious party foods that teenagers can enjoy, you will serve your own cause by showing your children and their friends that good food doesn't need to be boring. Don't call attention to the fact that the party treats are healthy, though. They are sweet, crunchy, and tasty; they don't need an explanation.

Some party food ideas (check Chapter 10 for these and other ideas):
- Tofu custard
- Spice cake (carrot or apple) with a special icing
- Oatmeal biscuits (no extra sugar)
- Apple cinnamon pie
- Fresh popcorn; liven the taste by sprinkling with Parmesan cheese
- Fruit–nut cocktails
- Smoothies
- Pumpkin cake
- Baked apples
- Carrot sticks and peanut butter
- Celery sticks stuffed with low-fat cottage cheese
- Skewered fruit and chunks of Cheddar cheese
- Homemade, no-sugar banana or blueberry sorbet
- Frozen banana ice lollies and crunchies
- Yoghurt freezer ice lollies

NUTRITIONAL SUPPLEMENTS

My work with several thousand patients has convinced me that a broad-based programme of nutritional supplementation is a good idea for adolescents and adults alike. Although my diet plan is designed to supply a complete range of nutrients, adolescents have special needs. They are in a period of rapid growth and emotional stress, and they may also be performing strenuous exercise. Inevitably, they are eating some junk food, full of anti-nutrients. For all these reasons, nutritional supplements are a good idea.

Here is a list of the supplements I recommend. The most important – because they are most likely to be deficient – are asterisked.

Vitamins

B VITAMINS

Thiamine (B_1)	10 mg
Riboflavin (B_2)	15 mg

Nicotinic acid (B_3)	100 mg
*Pyridoxine (B_6)	25 mg
Pantothenic acid	100 mg
*Folic acid	400 μg

I don't routinely recommend large doses of B vitamins. In addition to being unnecessary, they can make acne worse. Also I don't like to include vitamin B_{12} in multivitamin pills because a mixture of vitamins B_2, B_{12} and C and the mineral copper in the stomach can change B_{12} into a harmful substance called a B_{12} analogue that can actually interfere with the action of B_{12} in the body.

| *Vitamin A (as beta carotene) | 15,000 international units |

Beta-carotene has no known toxicity. The body changes it into active vitamin A, or retinol, at a controlled rate. I sometimes use retinol supplements; the indications for retinol are described later in this chapter.

| *Vitamin C | 1000 mg |
| *Vitamin E | 400 international units |

Vitamin C and vitamin E are anti-oxidants. They protect the body from the toxic effects of free radicals, chemicals that can damage tissues and cells. Free radicals are found in heat-damaged oils such as those used to fry or deep-fry any food. They can also be created when white blood cells burn off such poisons as air pollutants (the formaldehyde in new carpets and new clothes, fresh paint, solvents and cleaning solutions, car exhaust, certain types of glue, for example) or heavy metals that contaminate drinking water (cadmium and lead from water pipes, the mercury that leaches out of a fresh dental filling).

Minerals

*Magnesium	300–500 mg
*Zinc	15 mg
*Copper	1 mg
*Selenium	100 μg
Manganese	10 mg
*Chromium	400 μg
Molybdenum	400 μg·

The manganese dose may appear high, but manganese in pills is very poorly absorbed, and 10 mg is quite safe. The only danger with oral manganese supplements occurs in newborn infants, because they absorb it so readily.

I don't include iodine for the same reasons I don't like large doses of B vitamins – it is usually unnecessary, and it can make acne worse.

I also omit iron because it blocks absorption of zinc, copper and manganese. Iron deficiency can be a problem with teenage girls. They should be checked periodically, and if the level of ferritin in their blood is low or falling, then they should take a separate iron supplement: 20 mg chelated iron twice daily with food and 500 mg of vitamin C to enhance absorption. They should take this for three months or until the ferritin becomes normal.

Chromium and molybdenum are trace minerals, often lacking in our diet. Chromium plays a role in stabilizing blood sugar. Chromium deficiency may contribute to diabetes and hypoglycaemia.

EFAs

*Linseed oil	1 tbsp (15 ml) daily *or*
Cod-Liver oil	1 tsp (5 ml) daily *or*
Walnut oil	2 tbsp (30 ml) daily

HOW TO COPE WITH YOUR TEENAGER'S HEALTH PROBLEMS

Many of the health problems to which adolescents are prone are partly or completely rooted in nutritional imbalances or inadequacies. Acne, obesity, bulimia, fatigue, period pains, mood and behavioural problems, headaches, glandular fever, irritable bowel syndrome and sore throats can all be helped, and some can be cured, through proper nutrition. The bonus is that a healthy diet may clear up more than one problem – headaches may disappear along with acne, for instance. Good nutrition restores the body's systems to good working order, while medical treatment merely deals with a specific symptom.

ACNE

Acne is the single most common problem affecting teenagers. It is *always* caused by a biochemical imbalance in the body, and several reports show an association with a modern Western diet.[1] For that reason, proper nutrition can help alleviate it and may prevent it.

At 12, Lewis had oily facial skin with blackheads and a bumper crop of pimples; at 14, he developed serious acne. He told me that none of the lotions his friends used worked for him. When a dermatologist prescribed the antibiotic *tetracycline*, his mother refused to let him give it to Lewis. She told me that she had also had acne as a teenager and had developed a serious yeast allergy from the same antibiotic.

I explained that acne is caused by an overproduction of *sebum*, an oil produced by glands in the skin under the influence of hormones. When the oil is thick, it may become trapped in the pores, producing whiteheads. When sebum is exposed to air, it darkens, creating blackheads.

Skin bacteria break down the sebum into irritating fatty acids that produce red pimples and cysts. The usual medical treatment involves antibiotics to inhibit the action of these bacteria and lotions to peel off the top layer of skin and clear the pores.

Male hormones and stress can stimulate sebum production, as can deficiencies of zinc, vitamin A and vitamin B_6 (pyridoxine) or, according to some reports, too much iodine. Allergic reactions to foods also increase sebum flow in some adolescents. In my experience, the old notion that rich foods, sweets, chocolate and fats cause acne is valid in about 50 per cent of the cases.

I realized that Lewis needed to revamp his diet. I outlined a diet rich in vegetables and low in sweets, pastries and fatty foods. Lewis had no trouble dropping such fatty foods as bacon, fried foods and chocolate cakes, but he wouldn't or couldn't let go of his pizza and ice cream obsessions.

Lewis was taking a high-potency multivitamin. I had him stop it immediately. Most people think megadoses of vitamins help clear up acne, but some B vitamins can make it worse. I find that vitamins A and B_6 and zinc, without other Bs, usually work best.

But Lewis had normal blood levels of A and B_6, and normal levels of zinc in his hair and sweat, so I decided to explore the role of stress. While his diet changes had improved his acne, it invariably flared up again whenever he was under pressure. At such times, he also ate large quantities of ice cream. I wondered whether a milk allergy might be another culprit. I persuaded Lewis to stop eating or drinking milk and all other foods containing milk or milk derivatives for a full week. At the end of the week, he could eat and drink as much milk and ice cream as he liked for one day.

The first part of this treatment is *elimination*, when we see whether eliminating a specific food or group of foods improves an allergic condition. The second part is the *challenge*, when we see whether adding a specific food back into the diet worsens the allergy. To work well, the elimination must be complete. Lewis had to forgo milk, cheese, cream, ice cream, yoghurt, butter, and bread and cakes made with milk, milk solids or whey. He had to watch out for two milk proteins – *casein*, sometimes seen on labels as sodium caseinate, and *lactalbumin* – commonly used as food additives. Caseinate is used in margarine and non-dairy creamers.

Lewis's skin didn't clear up much on the milk elimination diet, but when he challenged it by stuffing himself with milk, cheese and ice cream, his whole face broke out in pimples. Subsequently, several weeks of a balanced diet that eliminated all milk products helped clear his skin up. That did it: Lewis was now convinced that milk products, including his beloved ice cream, were involved in making his acne worse.

But he would still break out when under stress – every exam at school gave him polka dots. I had to conclude that, although the dietary changes had helped, they couldn't completely clear up his condition. I decided it was time to see whether nutritional supplements would make any difference.

In my experience, the very best test for a nutritional need is simply to see how the body responds to a supplement. Would Lewis's stress acne respond to zinc? I suspected a daily dose of 20 mg would work – and it did. But I was reluctant to give him zinc alone, because it can induce other mineral deficiencies. So I switched to a multi-*mineral* supplement without iodine, which provided the following daily doses: 20 mg of zinc, 1 mg of copper, 100 μ (micrograms) of selenium, 10 mg of manganese and 200 μ of chromium.

EFA supplements help acne, too. Many adolescents with facial acne have dry skin on their legs. Linseed and cod-liver oil can help to shift the balance, drying their faces and oiling their legs.

A regimen for acne

Here are the things I advise my patients to do for acne:

- Follow my basic low-sugar, low-fat diet.
- Take 1 tablespoon (15 ml) linseed oil or 1 teaspoon (5 ml) cod-liver oil daily.
- Take 10,000 international units vitamin A daily.
- Take 20 mg zinc daily.
- Take 50 mg vitamin B_6 – *not B complex* – daily.

If there is no improvement after three weeks, eliminate *all* milk and milk products for two weeks. That means your teenager should avoid milk, butter, cream, cheese, yoghurt, ice cream, non-dairy creamers, margarine and any baked goods made with milk, milk solids or whey.

Sometimes higher doses of zinc and vitamin A are needed, but they should *only* be administered under the supervision of a doctor specializing in nutrition. Studies of nutritional supplementation for acne yielded the following results:

- *Vitamin B_6:* 50 mg a day prior to the start of periods diminishes premenstrual acne flare.[2]

- *Vitamin A:* 100,000 international units a day plus 800 IU *vitamin E* induces relief from acne within a few weeks. Maintenance on lower doses is effective.[3]
- *Zinc* in doses of 90–150 mg a day is as effective as antibiotics.[4]

EATING DISORDERS

Obesity

This is the number-one concern of adolescents, particularly girls. It's a threat to health and can be a threat to a teenager's self-esteem. Most people would say the cure is obvious: stop overeating. But eating too much is not usually the problem: The basic cause of obesity is probably lack of exercise. The *second* cause – and this may surprise you – is malnutrition. Or perhaps it would be better to call it 'undereating'.

Studies show that many obese children do not eat more than other children; in fact, many of them eat less. But fat children are much less active than their thinner friends. They play fewer games and compete in fewer sports, they sit more than they stand, they rarely jump around, and they walk when other children run. In swimming pools, they are frequently seen standing and talking!

Television in the home is a major contributor to the increase in obesity in children and adults.[5] TV viewing should be strictly regulated or it soon gets out of hand. It is too easy for your teenager to come home from school, flop down on the sofa, turn on the TV and watch it mindlessly. Kids in front of the TV sometimes seem to sink into a coma-like state.

I suggest that neither meals nor snacks be served in front of the TV. I also suggest no weeknight viewing except for school assignments and special events. For this reason, I am against separate TVs in bedrooms or kitchens. Daytime viewing on weekends should also be cut out.

Instead, encourage your teenager to get involved in some kind of after-school and weekend sports programme. If he's not on a school team, there may be community teams, swimming programmes or dance classes. If your teenager has not yet had his growth spurt and is too small to play regularly for school teams, help him find a sport he enjoys and can play well.

If you want your teenager to be active, you will have to become active yourself. You can jog or play tennis or squash with your teenager, and the whole family can cycle and play ball games. Long walks or weekend hikes are first-rate exercise, too.

Nutritional density: giving the body what it needs. Even though they eat fewer calories, people in Western societies today weigh more than their grandparents did. Why? We are less active than our forebears and the foods we eat actually contain *fewer nutrients per calorie* than the foods our ancestors ate. For example, we eat polished grains instead of brown rice, wholewheat bread and so on.

The nutritional value per calorie is called *nutrient density*.[6] Lean meats, eggs, milk, vegetables, nuts, seeds, poultry and seafood all have a high nutrient density – loads of vitamins, minerals and essential amino and fatty acids for each calorie. Sugar, foods in which the main ingredients are sugar and/or hydrogenated oils, and foods made with heat-damaged fats or refined flour products all have a very low nutrient density.

So two children might eat exactly the same number of calories, but the one on a diet of high-nutrient-density foods will be well nourished, while the one eating low-nutrient-density foods will be malnourished – and very possibly obese.

Why crash diets don't work. Dieting often makes the situation worse. When adolescents go on low-calorie diets, they eat much less of certain vital nutrients than they need; they become more malnourished. When they stop dieting, they go back to high-calorie but low-nutrient-density foods. The result is that they gain all the weight back, and they are still malnourished. When they go on another crash diet to lose the weight they have regained, they invariably lose less weight than they did the last time.

An interesting study with obese rats confirms the fact that each new crash diet results in less weight loss: Genetically obese rats were placed on low-calorie diets and lost weight. When they were then allowed to eat as much as they wanted, they gained weight. Each time they were dieted, they lost less weight than they had the time before, while each time they were fed as much as they wanted, they gained more weight than the time before. *The result was that, at the end of each recurrent diet, they were actually fatter than rats that had never dieted.* This happened even though they didn't eat more calories than the rats that had never dieted. Dieting actually slowed down their metabolic rates.

I strongly believe that the answer to adolescent obesity is not simply cutting calories. If overweight teenagers are going to lose weight permanently, they will have to become more physically active and begin eating high-nutrient-density foods.

I first saw Rebecca when she was 12. Her parents were both overweight, and she had never been particularly thin. But she had no serious problem until she began to menstruate at 10. After that, she began to gain weight, although she was eating just as she always had. The only change was in her activity; she had become much less physically active.

Becky was upset about the way she looked, and she became self-conscious and shy. She didn't have enough discipline to diet, though, and that ultimately proved to be her salvation.

I started by analysing Becky's and the family's eating patterns. Breakfast, generally cold cereal and milk, was rushed; there never seemed to be enough time to prepare a nourishing meal and eat it. Becky took a packed lunch to school, but she often didn't like it and simply drank milk instead. After school, she felt starved and would eat a cheese sandwich, another glass of milk and, often, a few biscuits. At dinner, she usually ate meat, potatoes and two vegetables, plus bread and butter and another glass of milk. The family didn't eat dessert, but in the evening Becky would watch TV and eat some sweet biscuits or cheese and cream crackers and have another glass of milk before going to bed.

Becky's major problem seemed to be her sedentary lifestyle, which involved her family as well. I recommended that, instead of TV-watching in the evening, the family go for a walk or do exercises together; I suggested they might even search out a nearby community centre swim programme. Exercising together would both make them more active and get them involved in doing things as a family.

The second problem was that Becky wasn't eating enough high-density food. Luckily, she wasn't a big junk-food eater either. Most of her calories came from milk, cheese and white flour. (In fact, I suspected a milk allergy might be the cause of her lethargy and nasal congestion.)

Finally, Becky ate too many of her calories late in the day or just before bedtime. As a result, she wasn't hungry in the mornings, and felt she could get by on a light breakfast and virtually no lunch. But by the time she got home from school, she was hungry and ate a cheese sandwich because it was quick and easy.

I recommended the following for Becky:

- No snacking after supper
- A big, nutritious breakfast
- A nutritious packed lunch at school (*see* Chapter 10 for breakfast and lunch recipe suggestions)
- Only two glasses of milk a day
- No cheese, white-flour bread or biscuits in the house
- Only high-nutrient-density snack foods in the house

Becky's interest in losing weight motivated her to follow my basic nutritional programme, which is not designed as a low-calorie weight-loss programme. Over a period of several months, she slimmed down considerably. She had more energy, and became much more physically active.

Bulimia

One of several serious eating disorders traceable to the malnutrition caused by dieting, bulimia is on the increase among teenage girls. It shows itself in a pattern of compulsive binge eating, followed by self-induced vomiting or the use of laxatives to remove the food quickly from the body.

Bulimia usually starts after a period of extreme dieting, and may also follow a period of anorexia (self-starvation). Sometimes it seems to the teenager to be an easy way to control weight. Soon, she (bulimia affects very few boys) becomes compulsive about that control and, paradoxically, her binge/purge cycle becomes uncontrollable.

Bulimics are often depressed, and some experts recommend psychotherapy. But Stephanie Dalvitt-McPhillips, an American therapist who suffered from both anorexia and bulimia as a teenager, has developed a different method to use with young people who haven't been helped by therapy.[7]

Dalvitt-McPhillips observed that episodes of bingeing always seemed to be preceded by crash diets of fewer than 1200 calories a day. In a controlled study of 215 bulimic students, she was able to produce rapid and permanent remission by having them consume a high-nutrient-density diet of at least 1400 calories a day, supplemented with a multivitamin–mineral tablet. The 200 extra calories a day were enough to prevent binges, and none of her subjects relapsed during the next five years.

Despite their binge/purge cycles, all the young women were slightly overweight when they started the treatment programme. On 200 extra calories of high-nutrient-density foods a day, they all lost weight.

Dalvitt-McPhillips's study appears to prove two important contentions:
• It's not how much you eat, but *what* you eat that determines what you'll weigh.
• Bulimia is not only psychological in origin; it is a biochemical disturbance that can be triggered by a crash diet.

The weight-conscious adolescent has to learn that the route to permanent weight control is through sound nutritional habits. Those who eat lots of vegetables, seafood and whole grains, and very little sugar, fat and white flour, will be slim without counting calories.

PERIOD PAINS

These are caused by an overproduction of certain prostaglandins, the chemicals that are the end product of EFA metabolism and that regulate every system in the body, including the immune system. The medical treatment is aspirin, or drugs such as paracetamol, which inhibit prostaglandin synthesis.

But drugs treat only the symptoms; the real cause of period pains (medically called *dysmenorrhoea*) is usually a deficiency of omega-3 EFAs. Magnesium deficiency can make the pains worse. *I have never seen a case of period pains that did not respond to EFAs and magnesium.*

I recommend the following:

• Follow my basic low-fat diet plan.

• For omega-3 EFAs, supplement with 1 tablespoon (15 ml) of linseed oil daily. Even better might be MaxEPA fish-oil extract, 2 to 6 g a day. Since too much oil could worsen acne, I always go for the lowest dose that will be effective.

• Supplement with magnesium, about 3 mg per pound of body weight. This is often extremely helpful.

RESPIRATORY INFECTIONS, SORE THROATS, COLDS AND FLU

Some children hardly ever get these irritating illnesses, while others are plagued by them. An occasional respiratory infection is normal at any age, and a healthy event in childhood. Most are caused by viruses, and in those cases, antibiotics are not helpful; in fact, they may even be harmful. Although in this age group some respiratory infections – bacterial sore throat ('strep throat'), bronchitis and pneumonia – may be caused by bacteria, most cases of bronchitis are viral in origin and don't warrant antibiotics. (Bacterial infections of the middle ear and sinuses may occur also. Fever and localized ear or facial pain are usually present.)

When antibiotics *are* used, there is almost *never* a reason to use anything but the old standbys: penicillin or erythromycin. I am appalled at the cavalier use of new broad-spectrum, superpowerful antibiotics such as amoxycillin (Amoxil) or cephalexin (Keflex) for simple respiratory infections. Their use encourages the growth of resistant organisms. They kill off health-promoting bacteria, especially in the intestines, encouraging an overgrowth of undesirable organisms, especially yeast. This is a *major* factor in promoting allergy. *It is no accident that the most allergic generation in history has been raised on antibiotics.* Several times a week I see a new patient whose allergies appeared or became much worse after a course of antibiotics.

Anti-yeast treatment to accompany antibiotics

If your teenager has to take an antibiotic, I strongly urge the following concomitant steps to prevent yeast overgrowth:

- *Acidophilus powder or pills.*
- If your doctor will cooperate, 1 million international units (two tablets) nystatin (Nystatin; prescription required) four times a day while on the antibiotic and for one week afterward. Nystatin should be taken on an empty stomach. It is not absorbed from the intestine and works as a kind of intestinal antiseptic against yeast. Its only side-effect is possible intestinal irritation.

Garlic oil can act as an over-the-counter addition to or substitute for nystatin. Capsules of this are sold in healthfood shops. The garlic is released in the intestine, so there is no breath odour.

Vitamins C and A

Some nutritional supplements are helpful in fighting *acute* viral infections. For the child with occasional mild infections (less than three a year), I recommend rest, chicken soup and T L C (tender loving care). For severe infections with fever, lots of aches and/or uncomfortable congestion, I find short megadose therapy with vitamins A and C helpful.

Vitamin C and immunity. Almost two decades ago, Linus Pauling began making controversial claims about the value of large doses of vitamin C in preventing and treating the common cold and other illnesses. He has since argued that adults should take several thousand milligrams of vitamin C daily for general health

While I respect Pauling's work, I don't recommend doses of vitamin C greater than 1000 mg a day for children, even adolescents, except under certain special circumstances. Colds reduce the levels of vitamin C in blood.[8] Several studies have shown that 1000–2000 mg a day of vitamin C can ameliorate the *severity* of colds but do not decrease the *number* of colds schoolchildren have each year.[9] Remember that 1000 mg of vitamin C a day is about 18 times the US RDA for teenagers (i.e. 55 mg) and *37 times* the UK RDA (27 mg). However, a daily intake of 1000 mg can be readily achieved by a diet rich in fruits and vegetables; it is not a true megadose.

Vitamin C supplements in the range of 1000–3000 mg a day improve wound healing and general immune response in tests of immune function in humans. This vitamin also has a direct anti-viral effect: it blocks the pathways by which viruses enter cells.

Vitamin C as a preventive and treatment. Vitamin C at a dosage of 1000 mg is a safe and reasonable (preventive) supplement for adolescents.

To *treat* severe colds, viral infections such as sore throat or bronchitis, and flu, I find megadoses of vitamin C very effective. If your child has fever and muscle pain and is home from school, I recommend the highest dose he can take: 1000 mg an hour, until he begins to get diarrhoea or loose bowels.

(Excess vitamin C causes diarrhoea because it draws water into the intestines.) This will establish his saturation point. Stop the vitamin C until the next day, when you should give him 1000 mg every two to three hours until his bowels again become loose. Stop the vitamins again until the third day, when you should give him 1000 mg every four to six hours. Maintain this dose until the cold is over, then gradually cut the dose back over two weeks to 1000 mg a day.

The anti-viral effect of vitamin C depends on getting the highest levels possible into the tissues. *Is it safe?* Very: not only against viruses, but also for acute allergic reactions. When should you *not* give vitamin C? If your child has kidney disease or is too sick to take food and liquid along with it.

Vitamin A and viruses.   For children over the ages of 10 vitamin A is also helpful with acute viral infections. It stimulates the immune system's killer T-cells, which kill viruses and cancer cells. The problem with vitamin A, though, is that it's *fat soluble*: it doesn't dissolve in water. For this reason, it accumulates in the body, and can become toxic. But toxicity depends on how much you take and for how long; I recommend very high doses but only for a very short time: 100,000 international units a day for three to five days. Larger or older adolescents weighing over 8½ stone (120 lb) can take 200,000 units a day for three to five days *maximum.*

Stop all vitamin A after three to five days. The levels in the body will slowly decrease. *Do not taper the dose off slowly; stop all at once.*

Note: I do not use this treatment with children under the age of 10, except in special circumstances. Nor should it be used if there's a chance of pregnancy; it may contribute to birth defects. *In any case, don't use this treatment more than once every 12 weeks.*

Some children have chronic or frequent respiratory infections or sore throats. This is neither normal nor desirable. Most of these children have been overdosed with antibiotics and are suffering from allergies and yeast problems. Often there are fatty-acid and mineral deficiencies. Loren's case is typical

Loren was a 15-year-old with a sore throat that had lingered for a year while she took antibiotics. Although the antibiotics had actually eliminated her original streptococcus infection, she still had white patches on her tonsils and swollen lymph nodes in her neck that looked like signs of bacterial infection. She had lost weight and was easily fatigued. She often felt dizzy and frequently missed school.

I told her parents that the first step in Loren's recovery was to stop the antibiotics. I put Loren on a low-sugar diet, with acidophilus supplements and nystatin to cut down on her intestinal yeast. To restore her immune system to normal, I prescribed:

Linseed oil	1 tbsp (15 ml) daily
MaxEPA (fish-oil capsules)	1,000 mg, 3 daily
Vitamin A	10,000 international units daily
Vitamin C	2,000 mg daily
Magnesium chloride	300 mg daily

multi-mineral supplement
Zinc	20 mg
Copper	2 mg
Selenium	100 μg
Chromium	0.2 mg
Manganese	10 mg

Over the next three to four months, Loren's sore throat disappeared. She gained weight and her vitality returned. This approach will help 80 to 90 per cent of teenagers with chronic or recurrent respiratory or throat infections. If it doesn't work completely, an allergy evaluation should be undertaken.

GLANDULAR FEVER

Glandular fever – medically called *infectious mononucleosis* – is common among teenagers. It used to be called the 'kissing disease' because it can be spread through saliva, but in fact, it is not generally understood how most cases are transmitted. It is caused by the Epstein-Burr virus (EBV), a member of the herpes virus family. EBV is possibly the most common human virus in the world. Almost everyone has been infected with it by the age of 35, but most never develop clinical mononucleosis.

The classic symptoms of acute glandular fever are severe sore throat, swollen lymph nodes (prominent in the back of the neck as well as the front) and severe fatigue with even mild exertion.

Although the throat may be full of pus, the infection is *viral*, not bacterial. Antibiotics should *not* be used: those with acute glandular fever are much more likely to have allergic drug reactions than those with other infections. Rest is important; the illness may last from two weeks to several months.

The vitamin C-to-bowel-tolerance regimen described on pages 167–68 is very helpful in glandular fever. In the convalescent phase, the following nutritional supplements are also helpful:

Magnesium   6 mg per pound per day (lower dose if diarrhoea occurs)
B complex   supplying per day: 50 mg vitamin B$_6$, 0.8 mg folic acid

If your child contracts glandular fever, he will be immune to it thereafter and cannot get it again. There are some people who develop a relapse of their old infection or who go on to develop a chronic illness called *myalgic encephalomyelitis* (ME). In most cases diagnosed as ME, the EBV is actually not the culprit, though. What's going on is obscure; the cause is either another viral infection or a more profound breakdown in immune organization. I have seen a few patients who developed acute glandular fever in adolescence who were never quite the same afterward: their initial illness was followed by chronic fatigue, dizzy spells, intermittent fevers, sore throats, swollen glands, muscle aches, depression, anxiety and the development of multiple allergies. Usually these patients don't seek medical attention as teenagers. They live with the symptoms and everyone thinks of them as troubled teenagers. The stress of adulthood makes them seek help.

My basic diet and the supplement plan for teenagers with chronic respiratory infections, outlined on pages 166–169, is quite helpful for many ME patients.

● *Magnesium* doses should be pushed almost to the point of diarrhoea – sometimes very high doses are needed to counter the fatigue. Doses of up to 1000 mg a day are safe.

● *Vitamin B$_{12}$* injections sometimes help dramatically. They may need to be given once or twice a week, 1 mg per dose. No toxicity has been reported with vitamin B$_{12}$, although some people feel *more* tired from it and shouldn't receive it. Positive effects are apparent within days – if they don't appear, the vitamin should be stopped immediately.

● Occasionally, high doses of the B vitamin *folic acid* are helpful. The US RDA for folic acid is 0.4 mg (400 µg) a day, but ME sufferers may need up to 10 mg a day to feel well. *Megadoses of folic acid can be dangerous, and this treatment must be supervised by a doctor who understands the risks and benefits.*

● *Iron* deficiency is not infrequent in ME. Your child's doctor should check the level of ferritin in his blood.

Viruses in the herpes family, including EBV, are nourished by an amino acid called *arginine*, which is found in high concentration in beans and nuts. (The cocoa bean, from which we get chocolate, is high in arginine.) But another amino acid, *lysine*, antagonizes arginine – prevents it from having its usual effect on a virus. For this reason, diets with a high ratio of lysine to arginine may offer some protection against recurrent herpes infections. It might make sense to have a youngster with acute glandular fever follow such a diet until he has recovered.

High lysine–low arginine diet

Note: This is *not* a good lifetime diet. It is recommended only for a few weeks.

EAT	AVOID
Eggs	Chocolate
Cheese	Nuts
Fish	Beans
Poultry	Tofu
Meat	

ME can be a disabling illness, and its treatment requires professional help. It is *not common* among teenagers; if your son or daughter is continually tired, there are probably other reasons for it.

FATIGUE

Fatigue is so common among teenagers, it's almost normal. If a teenager's fatigue prevents him from doing all the things he wants to, it's worthwhile making an issue out of it. The main reason teenagers get tired, in my experience, is that the nutritional demands of rapid growth and hormonal development are not met by their terrible diets. My basic diet plan has brought more than a few kids back to life.

Iron deficiency can cause fatigue long before it causes anaemia, so iron should be checked out. For a menstruating girl, or for a teenager who eats little meat, it's a good idea to test for iron deficiency. A blood-ferritin test measures the level of an iron-transporting protein. Low ferritin can reveal iron deficiency before a blood count does.

Aside from iron, the most useful dietary supplements are:

Magnesium	3 mg per pound per day
B complex	
Vitamin B_1 (thiamin)	15 mg
Vitamin B_6 (pyridoxine)	30 mg
Folic acid	0.4 mg

To treat a tired teen whose fatigue is food-based, I recommend my basic diet plan. I would also add a magnesium supplement – 3 mg per pound per day – and a B complex multivitamin supplying about 15 mg of B_1 and twice as much (30 mg) of B_6.

HEADACHES

The world's oldest complaint comes in three varieties: *tension, migraine* and *sinus.*

Tension headaches

These originate in muscular contractions of the head and neck. They are often experienced as pressure around the forehead or top of the head that travels down the back of the neck. They may be caused by injury, poor posture, nervous tension or stress, or they may be a secondary response to migraines.

Training in muscle relaxation is very helpful in relieving tension headaches. So is a magnesium supplement. Magnesium deficiency makes tension worse in much the same way as it does period pains. I recommend magnesium in doses of up to 600 mg a day until the headache improves or your teenager experiences a loosening of the bowels. This is the signal that the body has reached its point of toleration. At that point, cut back the dose and continue until the headache improves.

Migraine headaches

Caused by the constriction and dilation of blood vessels in the *covering* of the brain, they tend to come on quickly and can be very severe, lasting for several hours or days. They're often accompanied by nausea, vomiting and an inability to tolerate bright lights. Migraines may cause secondary tension headaches, which can last for days.

Several studies have shown that *food allergy* is an important cause of migraine headaches, especially in children and teenagers[10]. Disturbances in the body's handling of *calcium*, and in the actions of *prostaglandins* are also part of the migraine syndrome, so the body's supply of calcium, magnesium[11] and EFAs[12] had a major effect on migraine headaches.

The most dramatic migraine case I've seen was Patrick's. I saw him first when he was 13. He had been suffering from severe daily migraines since he was eight. He had not responded to any changes in diet or to any of a wide variety of drugs he had been given. At times, the constant pain made him so depressed that he considered suicide.

Patrick had some other problems as well. He hadn't grown significantly in three years, nor had he yet reached puberty. His doctor consulted me because of some very strange blood test results: the fatty acid levels in Patrick's serum and red blood cells were totally out of balance with each other.

My diagnosis was that Patrick would require very large doses of omega-3

EFAs in the form of fish oil. I recommended 16 g a day of MaxEPA capsules. The result was remarkable: over the next few months, Patrick's headaches began to subside. As they did, we gradually lowered his dosage of MaxEPA capsules to 5 g a day. To everyone's amazement, within three months after treatment began, Patrick also began to grow and develop sexually. Within a year, he had caught up with his peers.

A year later, I read a report from the University of Indiana on the use of high doses of fish oils to treat migraine headaches. Patrick's case, obviously, was far from unique.

Note: I would not recommend very high doses of fish oils without medical supervision. But you can safely give any teenager with chronic migraine headaches nutritional doses of MaxEPA (about 3 g a day) or linseed oil (1 tablespoon/15 ml a day), as well as magnesium (3 mg a day per pound of body weight). If your teenager doesn't respond, then you should investigate the possibility of a food allergy.

Sinus headaches

Sinus headaches are almost always allergic in origin. The pain is concentrated round the eyes and in the cheeks; it may also travel to the back of the head. Sinus headaches are often associated with nasal congestion, and tend to be worse in damp weather. They may improve somewhat with decongestants or antihistamines.

Chronic sinus headaches are usually caused by an allergy to moulds in the air or to foods, or both. Airborne moulds are concentrated in damp places such as cellars, swamps and forests. They're also more prevalent during early spring and autumn, especially when the humidity is high. Mould counts go up dramatically just before a storm.

Mould allergy usually requires treatment by a good allergist, but you can help relieve your teenager's sinus headaches by eliminating foods containing moulds and the moulds' close cousin, yeast.

- *Sugar* feeds yeast; your teenager should not only avoid table sugar and sweets, but also natural sugars found in fruits, fruit juices, milk and products made from flour, such as bread and biscuits.
- *Bread, cheese, prepared foods* such as soups that contain yeast or yeast extract, and *vitamins* made from yeast.
- *Fermented foods.* Yeast activates fermentation to produce alcohol and vinegar. Hidden sources of alcohol include cough syrups and vanilla extract. Vinegar is found in commercial sauces, ketchup, mayonnaise, salad dressings, soy sauce, and in sauerkraut and other pickled vegetables. Read all product labels for ingredients.
- *Naturally occurring yeast* and *mould* abound on the skins of some fruits, vegetables, seeds, peanuts and so on. Avoid dried fruit and commercial fruit

juices – apple juice is so yeasty that, untreated, it will ferment in a day or two at room temperature. Peel all root vegetables and remove the outer leaves of lettuce and cabbage. Nut butters are OK, but watch out for peanuts (especially prone to the cancer-causing mould aflatoxin) and other shelled nuts.

What's allowed then? Meat, fish, poultry, eggs, all fresh vegetables (except mushrooms), rice, potatoes, oats, rice cakes, nut butters.

You can decrease the growth of yeast in the intestine with either of the following natural substances:

• *Acidophilus.* Freeze-dried varieties are available from healthfood shops. Take ½ teaspoon (2.5 ml) a day before eating.
• *Garlic oil.* Do *not* use deodourized garlic oil. A good choice is natural garlic capsules, which are rich in the yeast-killing compound allicin. Take 9 to 12 capsules a day. Sometimes, when this treatment is started, the allergic symptoms worsen for a few days and then start to improve.

As soon as your teenager's symptoms start to clear up on any of the above, you can gradually reintroduce – one at a time – to your teenager's diet the foods that have been removed: nuts, seeds, fresh fruit, milk. Then begin to introduce vinegar, bread and cheese. Continue to avoid only those foods that bring on the headaches.

If the symptoms don't improve after two weeks with this treatment, you may need to consult a doctor who understands yeast allergy.

Bonus: This treatment may also aid migraine sufferers.

Prevent yeast problems before they start Be careful about exposing your youngster to antibiotics and sugar. If, for some reason, antibiotics are necessary, follow the treatment with two weeks of:

• *Acidophilus:* ½ teaspoon twice daily
• *Garlic oil:* three capsules of natural garlic with each meal
• Or have your doctor prescribe *oral Nystatin.*

IRRITABLE BOWEL SYNDROME

Irritable bowel syndrome, which produces abdominal pain, bloating, constipation, diarrhoea and, sometimes, mucus in the stool, is usually attributed to anxiety. It is the commonest intestinal disorder in the West, and usually begins in adolescence. It can certainly produce an irritable teenager, and severe cases can be disabling. My experience is that anxiety generally does play a small but definite role, depending on how severe the stress is. Some other factors are always worth searching for.

Abnormal intestinal flora or fauna

Common to two-thirds of irritable bowel syndrome cases is an abnormal level of intestinal flora or fauna, including a lack of healthy bacteria and an overgrowth of yeast or the presence of parasites. Treatment can produce dramatic relief.

Questions to ask: Has the teenager been treated with antibiotics? This, you will recall, can lead to a yeast overgrowth. Are there signs of yeast overgrowth, such as a rash around the anus or, in a girl, a vaginal discharge?

Has the teenager travelled to any parts of the world where he could pick up parasites? Has he gone camping in the mountains? Clear, beautiful mountain streams are often contaminated with the common parasite *Giardia lamblia*. Children are especially prone to intestinal infection by this parasite, which causes a mucus diarrhoea, abdominal pain and weight loss in its acute stages but may cause constipation and 'wind' in the chronic phase.

It's not easy to diagnose intestinal parasites, because stool samples are often misleading. The most reliable method I've found is the Bueno–Parrish Method, published in the *American Journal of Proctocology, Gastroenterology and Colon and Rectal Surgery* in 1981.[13]

Food allergy or food intolerance

These are present in almost all cases, but the standard diets don't take this into account.[14] The major offenders are dairy products, glutenous grains such as wheat, oats, barley and rye; and yeast- and mould-containing foods. Also important are fruits, nuts and beans.

By far the most common allergy is to *milk*. There are two kinds of milk intolerance: *lactose intolerance* and *milk-protein allergy*. Lactose (milk sugar) intolerance is created when there aren't enough enzymes in the intestine to break down lactose. Instead, intestinal bacteria break it down, making lactic acid that irritates the intestine, producing abdominal pain, 'wind' and diarrhoea. Lactose intolerance may be inherited, or it may develop when some other illness, such as infection, destroys the enzymes that break down lactose.

Since there is more lactose in whole milk or cream than in hard cheese, young people with lactose intolerance may be able to tolerate cheese.

Milk-protein intolerance is an allergic reaction to one of the proteins found in milk, and may show up also as a severe intolerance to cheese. Symptoms range from itching, wheezing and headache to abdominal pain, 'wind' and constipation or diarrhoea. Lactose intolerance, by making the intestine more porous, may itself cause milk-protein allergy and possibly other food allergies as well.[15]

Questions to ask: Is the teenager allergic? Does he or she have hay fever or asthma, nasal congestion, skin rashes or itching?

Overproduction of prostaglandins and calcium-generated spasms

These spasms have nothing to do with how much calcium your teenager consumes; they are caused by magnesium deficiency. Prostaglandin over-production, of course, is an imbalance caused by an EFA deficiency. I often find deficiencies of omega-3 EFAs and magnesium in young people with irritable bowel syndrome. Together, they contribute to the severity of the symptoms.

Questions to ask: Are there signs of an essential fatty acid deficiency, such as dry or rough skin, brittle nails or period pains? Are there signs of magnesium deficiency, such as muscle spasms and/or twitches?

Fourteen-year-old Wade provides a good illustration of how to track down the many causes of irritable bowel syndrome. For three years, ever since an acute illness diagnosed as food poisoning, he had suffered from chronic diarrhoea and abdominal pain. Wade's doctor had treated the food poisoning with an antibiotic, and although Wade's fever had subsided, the accompanying diarrhoea became worse.

When Wade tested positive on a lactose tolerance test, his doctor put him on a low-lactose, milk-free diet, but he didn't really improve. Although he took large quantities of anti-diarrhoeal and anti-spasmodic drugs every day, he could not fight off his symptoms.

I learned that Wade had done a lot of skiing in the Rockies and that as an infant he had frequently been given antibiotics for ear infections. As a child, he had suffered from hay fever and mild asthma, but had outgrown the latter.

I started Wade on an elimination diet that involved avoidance of milk, gluten, yeasts and moulds. This reduced his symptoms by 70 per cent, allowing a 50 per cent reduction of medication. But we found that if he deviated from the diet at all, he would come down with severe abdominal pain.

We added acidophilus. Wade reported three bad days, and then began to improve somewhat. He was able to stop his medication completely.

When we added linseed oil and magnesium, no immediate change was apparent, although Wade's hair became less dry.

A parasite exam revealed cysts of *Giardia lamblia* parasite, which is common in the Colorado mountains. We treated this condition with the drug metronidazole for seven days.

Now Wade's food tolerance began to improve; he was able to eat fruits, nuts and grains. Milk, however, remained a problem. A skin test showed that

Wade was allergic to milk protein, so we began a series of desensitizing injections.

Wade was by now virtually problem free. As a bonus, the following spring his hay fever was better than it had ever been.

Wade's story shows how complex the causes of irritable bowel syndrome can be. Here we had a young teenager who, as a child, had had allergies and had been deficient in omega-3 EFAs. His allergies led to recurrent ear infections, which were treated with antibiotics. The antibiotics, in turn, produced a yeast overgrowth that led to a yeast allergy that manifested itself in mild asthma and worse hay fever. To cap all this, Wade picked up a *Giardia lamblia* infection that produced acute gastro-enteritis, which left him with a lactose intolerance. The *Giardia lamblia* was misdiagnosed as food poisoning and treated with antibiotics, which brought back the yeast overgrowth.

Wade's intestines were now inflamed; the yeast overgrowth added to the inflammation and activated the *Giardia* infection. (It's known that *Candida*, the intestinal yeast, stimulates *Giardia* growth.)

With this series of events, intestinal function breakdown was inevitable, and with it, new food allergies developed.

What was the cause of Wade's irritable bowel syndrome? Pick something – anything – from the list above, and you'll be on the right track.

Fatigue, headache and irritable bowel syndrome often occur together. Consequently, their nutritional roots are often the same. They can be associated with anxiety, depression and emotional stress. If you're concerned about them, read the next section very carefully.

BEHAVIOURAL AND ACADEMIC PROBLEMS

The various pressures on your teenager – hormonal, social, academic, athletic – can produce reactions ranging from problems in concentrating on schoolwork to confusion, anxiety, depression and aggression. Usually, such problems are temporary, but if they persist, it's time for concern. If your teenager's schoolwork deteriorates, if he has trouble sleeping at night or suddenly loses weight, if he starts to withdraw from friends and school activities, if he becomes involved in drug or alcohol abuse or gets into trouble with the police, if he is fatigued or has headaches or abdominal pain as well, you will need to take action.

Many of these problems have underlying nutritional causes, but before we explore those, you will need to ask yourself whether you are giving your child plenty of nurturing attention. Adolescents need that if they are to give their best in school, in their social lives or in sports.

Now that most parents work, time for children must often be consciously scheduled, as it may also need to be if you have more than one child. Give each child just a few minutes of undivided attention each day – that's usually all a teenager needs.

The nutrition connection

There is no question that nutrition can be an important factor in a broad range of behavioural problems. Sociologist Stephen Schoenthaler has demonstrated that dietary changes as simple, in many cases, as replacing fizzy drinks with orange juice, can significantly decrease aggressive behaviour among boys held in juvenile detention centres.[16]

In most cases, I would expect my basic low-fat, low-sugar, high-fibre diet plan, with linseed oil (or cod-liver or walnut oil) and magnesium supplements, to help teenagers with concentration, depression or poor impulse control. The brain contains a high concentration of omega-3 EFAs; they are important for the normal activity of nerve tissue.

But sometimes a broader programme of nutritional supplementation is necessary. Two key elements are B vitamins and amino acids.

The brain uses B vitamins for building neurotransmitters and for providing energy. A combination that can significantly affect concentration, memory, and mood in some teens consists of:

B_6 (thiamin)	25 mg daily
B_6 (pyridoxine)	50 mg daily
Folic acid	0.4 mg daily
B_{12}	1 mg daily in tablets that dissolve under the tongue

Amino acids are the building blocks of protein. In the body, proteins are used to make everything from cell receptors to the neurotransmitters that carry messages from brain cell to brain cell. Most youngsters consume a lot of protein, so we don't usually have to worry about amino acid deficiencies. But when I studied a number of emotionally troubled adolescents who were eating high-protein diets, I found that, contrary to expectation, many of them were excreting very small quantities of amino acids in their urine.

I suspect that, in such cases, one or more food allergies are interfering with the proper digestion of protein, and that means that the formation of vital neurotransmitters may be impaired. Since our thoughts and feelings travel over neural (nerve) circuits, anything that impairs neurotransmitter formation is going to affect deeply how we think and feel, as well as how we behave.

Taking amino acids as supplements may have a noticeable effect on levels of neurotransmitters in the brain, and so can help relieve symptoms ranging from difficulty in concentration to depression and other behavioural problems.

A variety of supplements can affect memory and concentration:
- *Choline.* This amino acid is used by the brain to make acetylcholine, the key neurotransmitter involved in memory. Choline supplements improve memory in humans and animals. Choline is normally found in such foods as liver, eggs, oatmeal, tofu, lentils and split peas.

Supplements of 1000 mg a day are totally safe, *except during pregnancy.* Choline may be taken as plain choline capsules or as lecithin capsules (phosphatidylcholine). A good dose of phosphatidylcholine is 1000 mg three or more times a day. (Lecithin capsules comprise less than one-third choline.)
- *Pantothenic acid.* The body also uses this B vitamin to make acetylcholine. Pantothenic acid is found in liver, kidneys, oatmeal, brown rice, lentils, tofu, broccoli, mushrooms, avocado pears, cabbage, peas, cauliflower, trout and dark-meat turkey.

High doses of pantothenic acid improve wound healing and work with choline to enhance mental concentration. There are *no* side-effects. Doses of 500 mg two to three times a day are always well tolerated.
- *Glutamine.* This is an amino acid that enters the brain rapidly and is used as fuel. It is also converted to glutamic acid, an amino acid that stimulates the brain's response to acetylcholine. Glutamine should *not* be given to children with seizure disorders or liver disease; otherwise it is very safe. The dose is about 350 mg a day.

Depression   Don't try to treat a depressed teenager by yourself. *Professional guidance is essential.* Four amino acids used by the brain in making neurotransmitters may be helpful in the nutritional treatment of depression: tryptophan, tyrosine, phenylalanine and methionine. But their use is quite tricky – they should be given *only* under the guidance of a psychiatrist or doctor familiar with their vagaries.

The allergy connection

If you've read this book through, it won't surprise you to read that allergies to foods, moulds and yeast can play major roles in causing and sustaining behavioural problems in adolescents.[17]

If your child has difficulty concentrating in school and does not respond to a regimen of amino acids and pantothenic acid, suspect allergy, especially to foods or moulds, and provide some therapy accordingly. (See above, pp. 172–174 under 'Headaches'.)

More serious behaviour problems in teenagers can also be linked to food allergy, yeast infection, poor diet and nutritional deficiencies. In such cases, a stable, supportive family can be crucial to the success of nutritional therapy. Unfortunately, such was not the case with Terry.

When I first met Terry, she was a confused 15-year-old whose parents were divorced. Her mother had become a prostitute, and Terry lived with her father and stepmother.

Essentially, Terry had a bad self-image. Because she wanted to be liked, she was easily influenced by her peers. She smoked heavily and drank lots of coffee. She also ate a nutritionally deficient diet.

In my office, she showed signs of immaturity. She giggled a great deal and could not sit still. She was doing very poorly in school and was subject to mood swings, including depression and irritability. To add to her problems, she had acne, although fortunately it was mild.

Over the years, Terry had been given a lot of antibiotics for sore throats, bronchitis and hay fever. Her blood tests showed a vitamin B_6 deficiency.

I had many threads to weave with Terry. I got her to agree to drink less coffee, eat fewer sweets and take the nutritional supplements I find helpful with distressed adolescents:

B complex	supplying 50 mg per day of vitamin B_6
Vitamin E	400 international units
Vitamin C	1000 mg
Magnesium	400 mg
Zinc	20 mg
Copper	1 mg
Manganese	10 mg
Selenium	100 μg (micrograms)
Chromium	400 μg
Linseed oil	1 tbsp (15 ml) (or 1 teaspoon/5 ml cod-liver oil or 2 tbsp/30 ml walnut oil)

Terry's father reported that she was far less twitchy on these supplements, but I didn't notice any significant change in behaviour on her next visit to my surgery. Because of her long history of antibiotic use and because her skin tests showed allergies to several yeasts and moulds, I recommended that she go on a yeast-free diet and that she use the yeast-killing drug nystatin.

Terry had a remarkable response to nystatin. During her next visit she no longer giggled, and she could sit still! There was also a significant change in her behaviour at home and in school.

Sadly, though, after a few weeks Terry stopped taking the nystatin. She found a new boyfriend and started smoking and drinking coffee again, and this led to a relapse. Soon after, she ran away from home.

When she was found and brought back, her father had her committed to a psychiatric hospital. I discussed her case with the attending physiciatrists and they agreed to test nystatin's effects on her. First, they began a month of observation to get a baseline analysis of her negative and self-destructive behaviour. Then they restarted her on the nystatin and reported that they had observed measurable improvements in her behaviour.

You may have noticed that I treated Terry's behaviour problem in almost exactly the same way as Loren's sore throat. That was no accident; it underlies the most important message in this book. As said on page 1, children have a remarkable ability to heal themselves; doctors and medications do not make them better. When a child is given penicillin for a sore throat, it is not penicillin that cures the infection, it is the child's immune system. The penicillin may make it a bit easier, but controlled studies have failed to show that the child gets better much faster with penicillin than without it. Similarly, nutrition does not cure disease. Optimum nutrition merely allows a child to heal himself as effectively as possible.

Most chronic illness, from chronic sore throat to headache and anxiety, results from a child's inability to heal himself. In our culture there are a number of stumbling blocks to effective self-healing. Some of these are so common that they affect most sick children: dietary deficiencies of omega-3 EFAs and magnesium, plus excessive consumption of sugar, refined carbohydrates and processed fats and oils. Various mineral deficiencies (iron, copper, zinc, selenium) are close behind.

Excessive use of antibiotics is another huge barrier to self-healing; it causes a loss of normal bacteria and an overgrowth of undesirable micro-organisms, especially yeast. Yeast overgrowth can lead to yeast allergy.

Correcting EFA or mineral deficiencies or yeast overgrowth problems does not cure disease; it allows your child to heal himself by removing the impediments that were making him sick. It doesn't matter what the particular illness is – *we're not treating the illness, we're treating the child.* If you understand this principle, the next chapter should come as no surprise. The same nutritional aids that allow your child to bounce back from childhood illness also help to prevent the common degenerative diseases of adulthood.

How Power-Packed Nutrition
Creates Immunity for Life

9

Health is more than the absence of disease. Health is the vitality that confers resistance to chronic disease. Nowhere is this easier to see than in the face of a happy child at play. Her vitality is nourished by lots of love and imaginative play; optimum nutrition will help her to maintain it into adulthood. A wonderful dividend of the nutrition plan in this book is that, in addition to helping you raise a disease-resistant child, it will help your child avoid the most common and dangerous degenerative diseases of adulthood.

Each age has its characteristic diseases. In childhood, infection and allergy are the commonest; they represent a malfunction of the immune system. In allergy, some immune responses are abnormally hyperactive, whereas in chronic infection, other immune responses are not active enough. It is important to understand that these two conditions often occur together. The problem is not usually that the immune system as a whole is too strong or too weak; rather, it is *disorganized*.

Immune disorganization contributes to some of the commonest and most lethal adult diseases. On one side, there are the diseases of inflammation: arthritis, colitis, multiple sclerosis and autoimmune diseases such as lupus. Sadly, all these disorders, in which the body's immune system turns against the body's own organs, are increasing among young adults at an alarming rate.

On the other side lies cancer, which, until AIDS, was the most feared disease of this century. In cancer, the immune system fails to destroy defective cells that form continuously in the body. Normally, patrolling white blood cells zap them before they gain a foothold; when the immune response fails, the defective cells grow unchecked.

It is worth noting that people with cancer are more likely to develop autoimmune disease, and vice versa. As diseases of immune disorganization, cancer and inflammatory diseases are the degenerative adult counterparts of chronic infection and allergy. Throughout life, there is no environmental factor more important to a well-regulated immune system than a diet that properly balances EFAs and the co-factor nutrients that govern their metabolism.

The largest group of adult diseases is those that primarily affect circulation: atherosclerosis, hypertension (high blood pressure) and diabetes. All these conditions damage the body by decreasing blood flow to vital organs. Fatty deposits, thickened linings and overgrowths of fibrous tissue all narrow blood vessels in the heart, kidneys and brain. In diabetes, the major factor in circulatory damage is an excessive level of sugar in the blood; in hypertension, it is the high pressure within the blood vessels, causing them to become scarred and blocked. In atherosclerosis, the major factors are still controversial, but high blood levels of cholesterol and chronic psychological stress play important roles.

None of these disorders is primarily caused by impaired immune function, but they all involve the same derangements in cell chemistry that cause immune-system disorganization. If you look at the individual cells involved and at the prostaglandins they make – which, in turn, govern their growth and functioning – amazing similarities emerge among allergy, cancer and circulatory disease. The scientific evidence suggests that all of today's common diseases are caused by a common set of biochemical disturbances that have reached epidemic proportions in Western society. These disturbances produce different diseases in different people, depending on their inherited predisposition, their life experiences and the quality of their nutrition.

Chronic degenerative diseases don't just happen; they develop invisibly over the course of many, many years. In addition to helping you make sure you have the healthiest possible child, the nutritional guidelines I've given you in this book are designed to safeguard her from chronic degenerative disease as she matures. In this chapter, I will look specifically at three groups of diseases and pinpoint the scientific evidence that shows how my diet of high-fibre, low-sugar, low-fat, EFA-and-mineral-rich foods can protect against chronic disease in adulthood.

DISEASES OF INFLAMMATION AND AUTOIMMUNITY

A great deal of my clinical practice is involved with patients suffering from autoimmune diseases or chronic inflammatory conditions whose causes are as yet unknown to science. I've found that very often these conditions are accompanied by unsuspected nutritional deficiencies. In fact, it was through my work with such patients that I learned firsthand how important nutrition is to the practice of medicine. Working with them was the initial stimulus to do research on the therapeutic role of EFAs, magnesium and the anti-oxidant nutrients. Clinical studies by other researchers, epidemiological studies and animal experiments have all confirmed my observations. (Epidemiologists investigate the distribution of diseases in different populations.)

EFAs   Fat is an issue in most inflammatory diseases. Multiple sclerosis, for example, is associated with diets high in saturated fats.[1] In British studies, patients with multiple sclerosis[2] and rheumatoid arthritis[3] have consistently improved when saturated fats were removed from their diets. When essential fatty acids were *added* to their diets, they improved even more.[4] Several studies have now shown that omega-3 EFAs, in the form of fish-oil extract capsules, work especially well for arthritic patients.[5]

A study reported a few years ago in the *New England Journal of Medicine*[6] seems to explain why. EFAs, you will recall, are metabolized by the body into prostaglandins, the chemicals that regulate virtually every system in our bodies, including our immune systems. The omega-3 EFAs in fish oils, it turns out, block the formation of the particular prostaglandins that create inflammation.

In multiple sclerosis, on the other hand, plant-based EFAs, such as the omega-6s in safflower, blackcurrant seed and primrose oils, can alleviate some of the symptoms and their underlying biochemical abnormalities.[7]

While these clinical studies don't prove that EFAs can actually *prevent* immune diseases, some epidemiologic and experimental data suggest that they can. Autoimmune and inflammatory diseases are rare among populations whose diets are high in EFAs and low in saturated fats – as is the traditional Japanese diet. At the same time, the incidence of these diseases is increasing in industrialized nations whose citizens eat a lot of saturated fats and few omega-3s. In animal experiments, mice and rats bred to develop autoimmune diseases were fed diets rich in fish oils. The results? They either didn't get the diseases they were genetically programmed to develop, or they got very mild cases.[8]

Selenium   While data on other nutrients is skimpy, some interesting

Danish studies have shown that people with rheumatoid arthritis have low levels of selenium in their blood. Given selenium in supplements, some patients improve.[9]

ATHEROSCLEROSIS, HYPERTENSION AND DIABETES

All three of these diseases radically affect the circulatory system – they cause heart attacks and heart failure, kidney damage and strokes. Their nutritional antecedents have been extensively researched and, once again, fat is a crucial issue.

EFAs Almost everyone knows by now that atherosclerosis is associated with high levels of cholesterol in the blood. Many people, though, are not aware that the culprit is not so much the cholesterol in food as it is the saturated fats. High cholesterol levels in the blood, atherosclerosis, and hypertension (high blood pressure) have all been *independently* linked to a diet high in non-essential saturated fats. Omega-3 EFAs, such as those found in fatty deep-water fish such as salmon and tuna and in fish-oil extract capsules, lower cholesterol and triglyceride levels and blood pressure. What's more, they actually protect against the development of both hypertension and atherosclerosis. Omega-6 EFAs, found in vegetable oils such as safflower, blackcurrant seed or evening primrose oil, have a similar effect.[10]

How do EFAs achieve this magical result? By actually altering the chemistry of the body. Once again, it's a question of prostaglandins. Saturated animal fats found in red meat, poultry skin, butter and cream, or saturated vegetable fats found in palm or coconut oil, or *any* oil that, although it might have been originally unsaturated, has been wholly or partially hydrogenated, spur the production of prostaglandins, which makes blood thicker and more easily coagulated and constricts blood vessels. EFAs, both omega-3 and omega-6, have *exactly the opposite effect*; they trigger production of the prostaglandins that *enlarge* blood vessels and make the blood less sticky. A diet high in saturated fats is guaranteed to set up conditions that are just right for the development of atherosclerosis and hypertension. Replacing these fats with EFAs does just the opposite.

Salt Both epidemiological studies and laboratory experiments offer abundant proof that animals and people who consume a lot of sodium chloride (common table salt) are far more likely to have high blood pressure than those who don't. Since sodium chloride is universally added to manufactured foods in large quantities, as is the equally injurious monosodium glutamate, it's crucial to read labels carefully before using any food in a can, bottle or packet.

Magnesium and the fatty-acid connection   Magnesium is a key mineral in the prevention of high blood pressure. Doctors Burton and Bella Altura of New York's Downstate Medical Center have shown that animals fed a magnesium-deficient diet develop high blood pressure. The Alturas believe that magnesium deficiency lies behind much human hypertension as well. The catch is that, once you've got hypertension, magnesium alone won't do much good, because the changes in blood vessels are irreversible.

Magnesium can't protect you against high blood pressure if you eat a lot of saturated fat, either. Mildred Seelig, executive director of the American College of Nutrition, has observed that saturated fat actually blocks the absorption of magnesium from the intestines. But – you guessed it – EFAs *increase* the amount of magnesium you absorb from food or supplements.

Many studies support Seelig's observation. Animal studies, especially those of Dr Yves Rayssiguier in France, have found that magnesium deficiency raises the levels of cholesterol and total fat in the blood.[11] Studies of humans have shown that magnesium supplements raise the level of the 'good' cholesterol, high-density lipoprotein, or HDL, that protects against heart disease. What's more, magnesium deficiency can be found in the majority of patients with heart disease, diabetes and high blood pressure. It's not known whether the deficiency causes the disease or is caused by it.[12] The causes of heart and blood-vessel disease are complex, but it does appear that *a diet low in sodium chloride and high in magnesium and potassium will prevent hypertension and vascular diseases, especially if it is also rich in EFAs and low in non-essential fats.* These are all characteristics of my basic diet plan.

Fibre   Soluble fibres, such as those found in oats, beans, vegetables (such as cabbage) and fruit (such as apples), tend to lower both cholesterol and blood sugar. For this reason, Dr John Anderson of the University of Kentucky Medical Center has pioneered the use of low-fat, high-fibre, high-carbohydrate diets for diabetics. Fats can worsen such complications of diabetes as high blood pressure and atherosclerosis, and Anderson was dismayed at the amount of fat in the American Diabetic Association's recommended diet. His group has found that, in addition to lowering blood-sugar levels in diabetics, his diets reduce fat and cholesterol levels in diabetics and non-diabetics alike. They also stabilize blood sugar in people prone to hypoglycaemia, a drop in blood sugar that produces weakness, confusion and unconsciousness.

Soluble fibre achieves its effects partly because, unlike many nutrients, it is not absorbed through the walls of the intestine in its original form. Instead, bacteria metabolize it and transform it into short-chain fatty acids. These are absorbed through the wall of the large intestine and enter the blood, which carries them to the liver, the organ that makes cholesterol and blood fat. The short-chain fatty acids signal the liver to stop producing cholesterol and other fats.

In addition, fibre-rich complex carbohydrates take longer to digest than high-sugar, simple starches such as sweets or cakes. That means that high-fibre carbohydrates release sugar into the blood at a slow, sustained rate rather than all at once.

When Emanuel Cheraskin was teaching at the University of Alabama School of Dentistry, he measured his colleagues' blood-sugar levels several times a day for a month. When the dentists followed their usual diets, their blood-sugar levels fluctuated wildly throughout the day even though none of them was diabetic. But when they switched to a low-sugar, high-fibre diet, their blood-sugar levels stabilized.

Some scientists speculate that a low-sugar, high-fibre diet will actually help prevent diabetes and atherosclerosis even in people who are genetically susceptible to these killer diseases. Epidemiological evidence bears this out.[13] Why? Because a stable blood-sugar level requires less insulin. When blood-sugar levels rise, the pancreas releases insulin into the blood, which drives the sugar out of the blood and into the cells, which use it for energy. Over time, repeated sugar 'zaps' can exhaust a weak pancreas. In diabetes, the pancreas can't make enough insulin to keep blood-sugar levels down.

Insulin also stimulates liver and fat cells to make more fat. So when you eat a lot of sugar, you might as well be eating fat, too. A low-sugar, high-fibre diet avoids all these pitfalls.

Not all the epidemiological and experimental evidence supports the theory that fibre can prevent diabetes and atherosclerosis. But if diabetes can be treated with a diet that is typical of entire populations who seldom develop it, it seems reasonable that following such a diet from an early age could prevent some susceptible individuals from developing the disease.

Vitamin B₆ (pyridoxine) This is an important co-factor nutrient, enabling the body to metabolize EFAs into prostaglandins. Vitamin B_6 deficiency also worsens the effects of EFA deficiencies. Vitamin B_6 deficiency in experimental animals speeds the rate at which they develop atherosclerosis. In addition, animals with vitamin B_6 deficiency have high levels of a toxic amino acid, homocysteine, in their blood. In humans, high blood levels of this amino acid are associated with the development of severe atherosclerosis at an early age.

Whole grains are the best food source of vitamin B_6. Many people will need to take B_6 supplements to get the full amount they need: 10 mg or more a day, five or more times the US RDA.

Selenium   Heart-disease patients have lower levels of selenium in their blood than do healthy controls.[14] Depletion of selenium from the soil of much farmland in the United States has decreased the selenium content of grains, so that the American diet is marginally deficient. You can get the selenium you need – about 150 μg a day – from fish. If you don't like fish, you may need a supplement.

Copper   Most people consume less copper than the 1–2 mg daily US RDA. On the other hand, varying amounts of copper are found in drinking water, leached in from copper pipes.

Copper deficiency elevates cholesterol levels and weakens the walls of arteries. Experimental copper deprivation leads to abnormal EFA metabolism. A recent unpublished study of copper depletion in healthy young men was stopped when several of them developed heart problems.

CANCER

Cancer represents a failure of the immune system. Our bodies continuously produce small numbers of cancer cells, but usually our white blood cells promptly destroy them. When the immune system is disorganized, a person's susceptibility to cancer is increased.

Major cancers in the United Kingdom occur, in men, in the lung, prostate, colon/rectum, bladder and stomach, and, in women, in the breast, colon/rectum, uterus, lung and ovary; in both sexes, skin cancer is the most common, but in the majority of cases, it is highly treatable. With the exception of lung cancer, which is caused almost entirely by cigarette smoking and is rare in non-smokers, and skin cancer, which is directly attributable to overexposure to sunlight, all of these major killers are largely influenced by diet. (Even lung cancer is to some extent affected by diet.) The following guidelines are aimed at helping you reduce your child's risk of developing cancer at any time in her life.

Fat   As a step toward reducing the frequency of colon, prostate, breast, uterine and ovarian cancers, the National Research Council of the US National Academy of Sciences recommended in 1982 that people cut their fat consumption by 25 per cent. These recommendations were based on the results of both animal experiments and epidemiological studies. The latter consistently show that breast, colon and reproductive-tract cancers occur more frequently in population groups that eat high-fat diets than in those that don't.[15] Epidemiology alone can't establish cause and effect, because high-fat diets are also associated with many other factors that may contribute to cancer – pollution, stress and a decrease in breastfeeding among women. All these factors are consequences of industrialization. Hundreds of animal experiments in which rats fed both high- and low-fat diets are exposed to carcinogenic (cancer-promoting) substances have also shown that *the more fat in the diet, the greater the risk of cancer*. Moreover, a high-fat diet produces more and bigger tumours.

As we've seen, though, not all fats are equal – there are good as well as bad fats. The exceptions, of course, are the polyunsaturated omega-3 EFAs. These essential fatty acids have to come from food; the body can't make them. This, in fact, is why they are 'essential'. One particular omega-3 EFA – eicosapentaenoic acid (EPA) – is found in the oil of such cold-water fish as mackerel, salmon and sardines, who derive it from the plankton on which they feed.

A number of epidemiological studies have shown that when people consume a lot of EPA, they have low rates of breast cancer. This is true of Eskimos who still eat the traditional diet, high in oily northern fish that are loaded with omega-3 EFA-rich fat. Experiments have shown that omega-3 EFAs can protect against breast and colonic cancers in animals.[16]

Fibre Tribal black South Africans who eat a traditional diet rich in roots and vegetables rarely get colon cancer. But as they move to the cities, they change their diets, eating less fibre and more fat and sugar. The more closely their diet matches that of white South Africans, the higher their rate of colon cancer. Exactly the same is true of black and Puerto Rican populations in the United States.[17] In animal experiments, rats fed tumour-promoting chemicals developed fewer colon cancers when bran was added to their diets. The protective ingredient here is insoluble fibre of the kind found in whole wheat and crunchy vegetables.

Seed foods These are the seeds of plants, such as rice, maize (sweetcorn) and beans. Dr Walter Troll, professor of environmental medicine at New York University School of Medicine, has described a low rate of colon, breast and prostate cancer in populations consuming large amounts of such foods. He thinks that enzymes contained in seeds inhibit tumour development.

Other compounds in seed foods, called lectins, may also protect against cancer by stimulating immune response in the intestinal tract. They probably do this by triggering the multiplication of such lymphocytes as killer and helper T-cells, which can kill tumours themselves or direct the production of antibodies against them. (For more on T-cells and the workings of the immune system, *see* Chapter 1.)

One Dutch study found that death from cancer in general – not just colon cancer – was *three times higher* in men on low-fibre diets than in those who ate a lot of fibre.[18] This study was carefully controlled to make sure that the effect could not be related to any other factor, such as high or low fat intake.

The anti-oxidants: vitamins A, C and E and Selenium As you will recall from Chapter 1, the anti-oxidant defence system helps protect lymphocytes from incinerating themselves when they burn off toxins and other invaders we eat or breathe in. It also quenches the 'sparks', or free radicals, that are given off when lymphocytes do their work and that, unchecked, can damage chromosomes, enzymes, and cell membranes. A great deal of experimental evidence suggests that the damage free radicals do can contribute to the development of cancer.

Epidemiological studies show that people who develop cancer in general, especially of the lung or oesophagus, consume fewer of these vital anti-oxidants and have lower levels of them in their blood. Other studies show that, in rats, anti-oxidants can actively prevent the development of several common kinds of tumours. When the anti-oxidants are withdrawn from their diets, the rats get more and bigger tumours.[19]

This chapter has had one very simple purpose: to assure you that the nutritional recommendations in this book have a double benefit. My diet guidelines were designed to help you raise children in the best possible health and with the strongest possible immune systems. As a very substantial dividend, this programme will also help protect your children against the major killer and degenerative diseases that wait to strike adults. Optimal nutrition in childhood is a gift that lasts a lifetime.

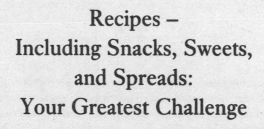

Recipes –
Including Snacks, Sweets,
and Spreads:
Your Greatest Challenge

There are dozens of cookbooks devoted to healthy, natural cooking. The purpose of this chapter is not to supplant them, but to establish some basic principles and to provide recipes for the standard meal plans. The recipes presented here are all you need to get started, but are in no way limiting. Your imagination and creativity can guide you well if you have a sound understanding of the principles explained below. I emphasize snacks, sweets and spreads because they present your greatest challenge.

BASIC INFORMATION

BREAKFASTS

Dinner would make the best breakfast for an active, growing child. Custom limits breakfast foods, however. Various cereals, breads and rolls, fruit, milk, eggs and smoked meats (sausage and bacon) are accepted as breakfast foods. While eggs are a good source of protein, vitamin A, iron and zinc, they are low in fibre and magnesium, and too high in cholesterol to be eaten daily – and recently they have been implicated in salmonella poisoning, which can be deadly for a young child. Served with whole-grain flours in pancakes or with whole-grain breads, it is all right to serve them up to twice a week as long as they are thoroughly cooked (at least 8 minutes boiling or poaching; frying will produce free radicals).

The rest of the meals will usually be built around cereals, and if whole grains – rich in fibre, protein and B vitamins – are used, the trick is to enhance their protein and mineral content with either milk products or seeds and nuts. So there are several recipes that present cereal-based high-protein breakfast foods.

DINNERS

These are usually the easiest. A hot meal combining a high-protein food with vegetables and starches is standard. The trick is to present less fat and more fibre and minerals than the usual British diet, and the key lies with beans (pulses) and seafood. Most of the dinner recipes provided are built on these as a major ingredient.

SWEETS

What creates a sweet? As the name implies, a sweet taste as well as a different texture (creamy or crunchy) and a pretty appearance. This can easily be accomplished with sugar and cream, but these ingredients are very low in nutrients. The challenge of sweets is to make them nutritionally rich, supplying, in particular, some vitamins and minerals missing from the remainder of the meal, and, at the same time, sweet and interesting in texture and appearance. Most 'natural food' cookbooks rely on honey for sweetness and vegetable oils or margarine for fat. This is not substantially different from using sugar and cream (at least cream and butter supply vitamin A). The composition of honey is not much different from sugar, although traces of some minerals and enzymes do remain in honey.

I have approached sweets from the following perspective: The main source of sweetness should be fruits – fresh, dried, puréed, concentrated – because fruits supply some vitamins and minerals that are often not easily obtained elsewhere. Examples: vitamin C in citrus fruits and berries, vitamin A in melon (cantaloupe).

For smooth texture, protein and additional minerals, either plain yoghurt or tofu, and for crunchy protein and minerals, nuts and seeds are called for.

Bulk and substance can be provided by whole grains, and eggs can contribute cohesion as well as their own protein and minerals.

For fat, my preference is a mixture of butter and linseed (or walnut) oil. Why? Linseed oil is an excellent source of omega-3 EFAs and has virtually no flavour. I do not like linseed oil for frying, because it oxidizes rapidly and the EFAs are destroyed. In baking, on the other hand, things are different. A hot oven has lost oxygen, and in the interior of baking bread or pastry, there is relatively little oxygen to destroy the oil. Butter need not be completely avoided by children. It contributes vitamin A and a pleasing flavour to the linseed oil.

A word about baking soda and baking powder. These are necessary for certain baked goods as they help dough rise. Baking soda is pure sodium bicarbonate; therefore, it adds sodium to the recipe. This is unavoidable and not a major concern if no other salt is added. On the other hand, baking powder is a mixture of sodium bicarbonate, calcium acid phosphate (as a stabilizer) and cornflour. Most baking powders contain sodium aluminium sulphate. Avoid these. Aluminium is a toxic metal that does not belong in anyone's diet, especially a child's. It can accumulate in the central nervous system and contribute to brain dysfunction. Some cases of Alzheimer's disease (senile dementia) are thought to reflect susceptibility to toxic accumulation of aluminium in the brain. Check your healthfood shop for an aluminium-free baking powder.

Aluminium can also enter food from aluminium cookware. The rate at which aluminium is leached from cookware depends on the acidity of the water and food, the duration of cooking and the presence of fluoride in the water. A study at the Institute of Fundamental Sciences in Hantana, Sri Lanka, published in the prestigious journal *Nature*, found that 1 part per million (ppm) of fluoride in water released 200 ppm of aluminium when boiled for ten minutes in aluminium cooking pots. That's 1000 times the amount leached out by non-fluoridated water. Prolonged boiling was capable of tripling the aluminium concentration. Since these concentrations of fluoride are found in some municipal water supplies, it seems prudent not to use aluminium cookware with fluoridated tap water. Highly acidic water, found in many wells, and acidic foods such as tomatoes also extract considerable aluminium. The only cookware we use in our household is cast iron, glass or porcelain, and occasionally stainless steel. (Teflon-coated aluminium cookware should be OK as long as the coating remains intact.)

STAPLES

In the section below, any products with an asterisk are generally available only in healthfood shops. Otherwise, all staples are available either in supermarkets or healthfood shops.

Grains and grain products

When you purchase grains in the supermarket, make sure the label reads 'whole grain', 'wholewheat' and so on. Refrigerate grains for maximum freshness.

- *Wholewheat flour*
- *Wheat flakes**
- *Wholewheat pastry flour**
- *Soya powder*
- *Soya flour**
- *Oat flakes*
- *Rolled oats* (for porridge)
- *Oat bran*
- *Wheat bran.* This can be found in bulk in healthfood shops.
- *Brown rice.* Most supermarkets stock long-grain rice. I prefer short-grain in general, although for rice pudding, the long-grain is more moist and tender. Purchase short-grain rice in the healthfood shop.
- *Barley flakes**
- *Wholewheat pita bread*
- *Pasta.* This comes in many colours and shapes. Experiment as you wish. Supermarket pasta made with semolina flour has slightly more nutrient value than that made with regular processed white flour. Those with added soya flour have more protein value. Whole-grain pasta has the highest nutrient value.

Dried pulses

Pulses (beans, peas, lentils, etc.) will keep up to a year. It is not necessary to refrigerate them, unless they have been cooked, in which case they will keep in the refrigerator for up to five days. Or store them cooked in the freezer in meal-size portions; they will keep up to three months. Look for pulses that are uniform in size and colour so that they will cook evenly. Avoid those that are dull looking, which indicates age, or have tiny pinholes, which indicates insect invasion. If you purchase canned cooked beans, try to find ones without added sodium. Rinse all canned beans well before use.

- Lentils
- Haricot beans
- Pinto beans (Mexican)
- Black beans
- Black-eyed beans
- Kidney beans
- Aduki beans
- Split peas

Many of these are now available from good supermarkets, and others can be found in healthfood shops. In addition, you can try looking in speciality grocers – e.g. Chinese, West Indian, Indian.

Oils

- *Olive oil.* If you use olive oil frequently, keep it out of the refrigerator, since olive oil becomes thick and cloudy when refrigerated. (It will return to its normal consistency after being left at room temperature for a few minutes.)
- *Linseed oil.** See page 13 for information on suppliers.
- *Unrefined sesame oil**
- *Walnut oil.* Available from good-quality supermarkets and grocers. Hold on to your seats when you see the price! This is just to be used as a delicious flavouring and for its good nutritional value.

Nut butters

- *Peanut butter (sugar-free)*
- *Sesame tahini.* Note that hummus ('sesame butter') is different from tahini. Hummus is made from ground sesame seeds, and chickpeas, oil and lemon juice and is much thicker in consistency, so it will affect the recipe. Sesame tahini is made from unroasted sesame seeds and is runnier.

These should be kept in the refrigerator to avoid rancidity. Be sure your peanut butter has no sugar added. Read the label. Remember that dextrose and corn sweetener are sugars. If you buy peanut butter freshly ground, be sure that it is refrigerated right away, since, without salt and preservatives, it becomes rancid quickly.

Nuts and seeds

Purchase nuts and seeds from a shop with a fast turnover, since they turn rancid quickly. Avoid those that look shrivelled, discoloured or mouldy. Store nuts and seeds in the refrigerator.

- *Sesame seeds*
- *Sunflower seeds (hulled)*
- *Pumpkin seeds*
- *Walnuts*
- *Almonds*
- *Hazelnuts*
- *Linseed**

Dried fruit

Purchase unsulphured dried fruit – that is, fruit that has not been treated with the toxic chemical sulphur dioxide to preserve the colour and soft texture. Unsulphured dried fruit will be darker and drier, but can be plumped up by soaking in hot water. It can be purchased in healthfood shops. Dried fruit can be kept in the freezer for months.

- *Raisins*
- *Pitted dates*
- *Dried apples.** If these are sold in bulk, they are much less expensive.

Seasonings and flavouring agents

- *Apple cider vinegar or rice vinegar*
- *Vanilla* and *almond extract.* Purchase pure extracts with no added artificial colour or preservatives.
- *Baking soda*
- *Frozen orange, apple and pineapple concentrates.* Concentrates are used as sweeteners. All frozen concentrates are found in the frozen foods section of the supermarket. They are what you would use to make fruit juice. Use them undiluted in the recipes.
- *Honey.* Be sure it has no added preservatives. Never give honey to a child who is less than one year old.
- *Soya sauce.* Be sure it contains no monosodium glutamate, caramel or added colouring. Kikkoman is a good brand. Purchase reduced-sodium soya sauce, if it is available. If your child is allergic to wheat, purchase wheat-free soya sauce.
- *Lemon juice.* Squeeze fresh.

Other staples

- *Tofu.* This comes firm, soft or silken. Use the kind called for in the recipe. If you can't find silken, use soft. Purchase it packaged in the dairy section of the supermarket. Tofu left sitting in water in the open, or stored in temperatures less than that required for dairy storage, may have bacterial overgrowth. Signs of spoilage are a bulging package and/or a smell like vinegar or sulphur. Store your tofu in the refrigerator in a container of water. Change the water daily. It should keep for three to five days. It will also keep in the freezer for up to two months, but will be spongier and more fragile.
- *Eggs*
- *Milk*
- *Plain yoghurt*
- *Frozen fish.* Fresh fish is preferable, but it helps to have some frozen on hand for last-minute meals.
- *Corn tortillas.* Ready-cooked tortillas are sometimes available in super-markets where Mexican foods are sold. Purchase those made *only* with corn, water and lime.

- *Jams and spreads.* Purchase those without any added sweeteners, including honey. Fruit-only spreads are becoming increasingly available; a good one is Whole Earth pear and apple spread (it keeps well).
- *Apple sauce.* Purchase unsweetened varieties.
- *Sugar-free ketchup* *
- *Desiccated coconut.* If you purchase it in the supermarket, be sure it is unsweetened. Read the label.

HOW TO OIL A PAN

To use as little oil as possible, put a bunched-up paper towel over the opening of your favourite cooking oil. (Olive oil is best for cooking.) Tip the bottle quickly upside down, then right-side up. Whatever small amount of oil is on the towel can be used to wipe the pan. Another idea: brush the pan with an oiled pastry brush.

For greasing baking tins for cakes and so on, a small amount of butter is fine. It contributes vitamin A and a pleasing flavour to the baked goods.

Most baking pans are aluminium or glass, but glass can be hard to find. Using a non-stick pan or lining the inside with greaseproof paper will keep baked goods from sticking and will act as a barrier between the food and the aluminium.

HOW TO COOK BEANS

Beans should be rinsed several times to get rid of grit and other particles.

All beans except lentils, split peas, aduki beans and black-eyed peas need to be soaked for at least three hours before cooking. (Soyabeans and chickpeas require overnight soaking.)

Since beans expand up to three times in volume when cooked, use a pot large enugh to accommodate their increased size when you cook them.

Most beans require two to four times liquid to the volume of beans.

To help get rid of the carbohydrate in the bean which causes 'wind', throw away the soak water and replace with fresh water to cook the beans. Also, after the first hour of cooking, replace the water again. You'll lose some nutrients but not many.

Although pressure cooking is faster, cooking beans more slowly (in a normal pot, that is) seems to result in greater digestibility.

A simple technique for determining that beans are cooked: Blow on a bean. If the skin pops, it's done.

Eating fresh beans is preferable to eating canned, since canned beans have added sodium. If you purchase canned beans, rinse them well to help get rid of the sodium.

Cooked beans keep up to three months stored in the freezer, and keep in the refrigerator for up to five days.

BREAKFAST: START THE DAY HEALTHY

JEFF'S BLUEBERRY WHOLEWHEAT PANCAKES

My son Jeff devised this recipe while making brunch for friends. It's become a regular Sunday treat.

MAKES EIGHTEEN 4½-IINCH (10.5 CM) PANCAKES
TIME SAVERS: The batter can be prepared the night before, if you like. In fact, it is even better if allowed to sit in the refrigerator for 3 to 6 hours before use. Alternatively, the dry ingredients (flour and baking soda) can also be pre-mixed and kept in the refrigerator until pancake time. Cooked pancakes can be kept in the freezer and put in a toaster or microwave.

6 oz (170 g) wholewheat flour
2 oz (55 g) soya powder
2 tsp baking soda
12 oz (340 g) fresh blueberries (see Note)
2 eggs
12 fl. oz (340 ml) buttermilk, or plain yoghurt
6 fl. oz (170 ml) water
2 tbsp (30 ml) linseed or walnut oil

In a large bowl, stir the flour, soya powder and baking soda until combined. Add the blueberries and mix until berries are coated with flour. In a medium-size bowl, beat the eggs; then add the buttermilk, water and oil, and blend thoroughly. Add the liquid mixture to the dry, stirring until combined. Don't overstir or beat the batter – a few lumps are not a problem, and too much mixing will result in tough, rubbery pancakes.

Heat large non-stick frying pan (*see* Note), then oil it lightly. Pour 2 fl. oz (55 ml) of batter on the pan for each pancake. Let the batter cook until bubbles appear on the surface and the edges look dry and begin to turn lightly brown. Then turn the pancake and cook about 2 minutes more.

If necessary, add small amounts of oil to the pan in between pancakes.

To keep the pancakes warm, preheat the oven to the warm setting and put the pancakes on a baking sheet in the oven as you go. If you stack the pancakes, put a cloth between them to prevent them from becoming rubbery.

If desired, top with apple sauce (an unsweetened brand), sugar-free jam, low-fat yoghurt or any of the sweet toppings on pages 238–239.

Note: Frozen blueberries do not work as well in this recipe as fresh. Blackcurrants can be substituted.

Using a non-stick frying pan will cut down on the need to use a lot of oil to make the pancakes, and they bake better on this type of surface.

SESAME WAFFLES

MAKES FOUR 7-INCH (18 CM) WAFFLES
TIME SAVER: The batter can be prepared the night before, if you like. In fact, it is even better if allowed to sit in the refrigerator for 3 to 6 hours before use. Cooked waffles can be kept in the freezer and reheated in a toaster or microwave.

4 oz (115 g) wholewheat flour
1½ oz (45 g) soya flour
1 tsp baking soda
3 tbsp sesame seeds
2 eggs
1 tbsp linseed or walnut oil
8 fl. oz (230 ml) buttermilk
3 tbsp water

In a large bowl, sift together the flours and baking soda. Add the sesame seeds. (At this point, I found it was perfect timing to start heating up an electric waffle iron.)

In an electric blender, mix the eggs, oil, buttermilk and water. Add the liquid ingredients to the dry, stirring with a few quick strokes till just mixed. Don't worry about a few lumps; it's better to underbeat than overbeat.

Lightly oil the waffle iron. Pour on 4 fl. oz (115 ml) batter per waffle. Each waffle takes between 3½ and 4 minutes to cook to a golden brown. To keep the waffles warm before serving, preheat the oven on the warm setting and put them on a baking sheet in the oven. If you stack the waffles, put a cloth between them to prevent them from becoming rubbery.

Top with sugar-free apple sauce, sugar-free jam, low-fat yoghurt or any of the sweet toppings on pages 238–239.

BRAN MUFFINS

These are a great non-sweet muffin. If you need a sweetener, top with a

non-sugar fruit spread or a sugar-free jam. Your children can help you coat
the raisins with the flour.

MAKES 12 TO 14 MEDIUM-SIZE MUFFINS

8 oz (225 g) wholewheat flour
1 oz (30 g) soya flour
2 tsp baking soda
¼ to ½ tsp ground cinnamon
4 oz (115 g) wheat bran
6 oz (170 g) raisins
1 egg
2 tbsp (30 ml) linseed or walnut oil
10 fl. oz (285 ml) buttermilk
4 fl. oz (115 ml) apple juice concentrate

Preheat oven to 400° F (205° C, gas mark 6), and lightly oil a bun tin or 14
paper cupcake cups.

In a large bowl, sift together the flours, baking soda and cinnamon. (If
there is any bran residue, add it back into the mixture. The sifting is designed
to make the muffins a little lighter; it's not done to remove bran.) Stir the
wheat bran into the flour mixture, then add the raisins and stir until the raisins
are coated with flour.

In a medium-size bowl, beat the egg with a wire whisk, then add the oil and
mix well. Add the buttermilk and apple juice concentrate, and beat
thoroughly.

Add the liquid ingredients to the dry all at once, stirring with a few quick
strokes until just combined. Don't overbeat or the muffins will be tough.
Spoon the batter into the lightly oiled tin or cups, filling each almost to the top
with batter.

Bake for 20 minutes, or until the tops of the muffins are lightly brown and a
toothpick comes out dry when inserted in the centre. Let the muffins sit in the
pan for about a minute, then carefully turn out on to a wire rack to cool for a
few minutes. Serve hot.

APPLE–COCONUT MUFFINS

MAKES 10 MUFFINS

6 oz (170 g) wholewheat flour
1 tsp baking soda
½ tsp ground cinnamon
3 tbsp flaxseed, ground (see Note)

1 egg
2 oz (55 g) unsalted butter, melted
2 fl. oz (55 ml) linseed or walnut oil
2 tbsp (30 ml) apple juice concentrate
8 fl. oz (230 ml) sugar-free apple sauce
2 oz (55 g) desiccated unsweetened coconut

Preheat the oven to 400° F (205° C, gas mark 6). Lightly oil 10 paper cupcake cups.

In a large bowl, mix the flour, baking soda, cinnamon and ground flaxseed. In a medium-size bowl, beat the egg, butter and oil. Then add the apple juice concentrate, apple sauce and coconut, and mix until well blended. Add the wet ingredients to the dry all at once, stirring just until the mixture is moistened. Don't overbeat or the muffins will be tough. Spoon the batter into the cupcake cups, filling each two-thirds full.

Bake for 30 minutes, or until the tops are lightly brown. The insides of the muffins will be slightly moist because of the apple sauce.

Note: Flaxseed can be ground in a coffee mill or nut grinder.

MUESLI I

MAKES 2 LB (900 G)

12 oz (340 g) rolled oats
4 oz (115 g) oat bran
1 oz (30 g) sesame seeds
1 oz (30 g) flaxseed
2 oz (55 g) sunflower or pumpkin seeds
4 oz (115 g) chopped walnuts
4 fl. oz (115 ml) apple juice concentrate
2 fl. oz (55 ml) linseed or walnut oil
1 tsp vanilla
1 tsp ground cinnamon
8 oz (225 g) raisins
2 oz (55 g) desiccated unsweetened coconut

Preheat the oven to 350° F (175° C, gas mark 4) and lightly oil two baking sheets.

Mix oats, oat bran, seeds and nuts in a large bowl. Combine the apple juice concentrate, oil, vanilla and cinnamon in a small bowl.

Add the wet ingredients to the dry, stirring until everything is well coated

with the oil mixture. Spread the mixture evenly on the two baking sheets.
Bake for 18 to 20 minutes, or until golden brown. Stir after 10 minutes.
Remove from the oven, and add the raisins and the coconut.

Store in an airtight container in the refrigerator. Serve topped with low-fat
milk or apple juice.

MUESLI II

MAKES 3 ½ LB (1.1 KG)

12 oz (340 g) rolled oats
12 oz (340 g) wholewheat or barley flakes
4 oz (115 g) oat flakes
4 oz (115 g) oat bran
4 oz (115 g) sunflower or pumpkin seeds
4 oz (115 g) chopped hazelnuts
4 oz (115 g) raisins
4 oz (115 g) chopped dried apples

Preheat the oven to 400° F (205° C, gas mark 6).

In a large bowl, combine the rolled oats, wholewheat or barley flakes, the
oat flakes and oat bran. Spread the grains out in a thin layer on 5 ungreased
baking sheets. (You could use fewer baking sheets by dividing the mixture
into five equal parts.) Shake each baking sheet so that you have an even
distribution of grains. Bake for 4 to 5 minutes, stir and turn the grains with a
fish slice, and bake them for an additional 1 to 2 minutes, until lightly
browned. Let them cool, then put them back in the bowl. When all the grains
have been baked, add all other ingredients and mix together.

Store in an airtight container in the refrigerator. Serve with milk or plain
yoghurt. Add fresh fruit in season.

STIR-FRIED TOFU

4 oz (115 g) firm tofu
1 tbsp (15 ml) olive oil
Sea salt to taste
⅛ tsp paprika

Slice tofu into squares about ½ inch (1.2 cm) thick. Heat olive oil in a
seasoned cast-iron pan and quickly stir-fry the tofu. Season with sea salt and
paprika, and serve.

SCRAMBLED TOFU

4 oz (115 g) firm tofu
1 tbsp (15 ml) olive oil
1/8 tsp turmeric
Sea salt to taste
1/8 tsp paprika

Mash the tofu. In a frying pan, heat the olive oil, and when it starts to sizzle, add the mashed tofu and, as you would with an egg, scramble with a fork or wooden spatula. Add turmeric for colour. Season with sea salt and paprika and serve like scrambled egg.

SUPER-NUTRITIOUS MAIN COURSES

LENTIL AND BARLEY STEW

SERVES 6

3 oz (85 g) dried lentils
3 oz (85 g) whole barley
6 oz (170 g) chopped onion
4 oz (115 g) chopped celery
1 tsp (10 ml) olive oil
2 1/2 pints (1.4 l) water
1/2 tsp rosemary
1/4 tsp thyme
1 bay leaf
12 oz (340 g) sliced carrots
12 oz (340 g) chopped potatoes
Salt to taste
Pepper to taste
4 oz (115 g) chopped parsley

Put the lentils and barley in a large bowl, and add water to cover. Pour off the water and refill the bowl. Do this several times until the water is clear. Drain and set aside. In a heavy pot large enough to hold the stew, sauté the onion and celery in the olive oil until the onion is transparent and soft. Add the water, drained barley and lentils, and herbs. Bring stew just to the boil, then turn down the heat, cover, and let simmer over low heat for 15 minutes.

Remove the bay leaf, and add the carrots and potatoes. Continue cooking until the lentils and barley are soft, about 30 minutes, stirring occasionally. When the stew is done, stir in salt and pepper to taste, then add the parsley.

LENTIL–NUT LOAF

This tastes great by itself or with a tomato sauce. It's also good cold, by itself or as a sandwich – great for school packed lunches.

SERVES 6

1½ oz (45 g) lentils
10½ fl. oz (300 ml) cold water
1 oz (30 g) linseed
4 fl. oz (115 ml) hot water
2 eggs
½ tsp (5 ml) soy sauce
¼ tsp thyme
¼ tsp rosemary
4 oz (115 g) chopped onion
4 oz (115 g) finely chopped celery
1 oz (30 g) chopped parsley
1 oz (30 g) sesame seeds
6 oz (170 g) nuts or seeds (sunflower seeds, almonds or pumpkin seeds), ground
2 oz (55 g) whole-grain bread crumbs (see Note)
4 oz (115 g) chopped walnuts

Rinse the lentils, removing any small stones. Put the lentils in a pot with cold water. Bring the water to a boil, lower the heat and simmer for 50 minutes, or until the lentils are soft.

Meanwhile, prepare the rest of the ingredients for the loaf. Put the linseed in a small bowl with the hot water. The seeds will absorb the water, forming a gel in about 20 minutes. This will help hold the loaf together. It will also provide a soft, crunchy texture, and the linseeds are high in EFAs.

Preheat the oven to 350° F (175° C, gas mark 4).

In a large bowl, beat the eggs, then add the remaining ingredients, including the cooked lentils and linseed gel.

Press the mixture into a lightly greased 9 × 5 × 3 in (23 × 13 × 8 cm) loaf tin. Bake for 1 hour.

Note: Make your own bread crumbs from homemade bread with a food processer or blender, or purchase bread crumbs that have no added sugar, salt, preservatives or colourings.

VEGETARIAN BURGERS

MAKES 10 BURGERS

Divide the lentil–nut loaf mixture into 10 equal parts and form patties that are 3 in (7.5 cm) in diameter and 1 in (2.5 cm) thick, or any size you like. Place the patties on a lightly greased baking sheet and bake for 15 minutes on each side at 350° F (175° C, gas mark 4). Enjoy the burgers with sugar-free ketchup and a whole-grain bun or pita bread.

SPANISH RICE AND BEANS

8 oz (225 g) dried pinto or kidney beans (see Note)
8 oz (225 g) short-grain brown rice
1 garlic clove, crushed
4 oz (115 g) chopped onion
5 oz (140 g) chopped sweet red pepper
2 tsp (10 ml) olive oil
14 oz (395 g) chopped tomatoes
2 fl. oz (55 ml) tomato purée
1 ½ tsp ground coriander
½ tsp ground cumin
Salt and pepper to taste

Soak the beans in 1 ½ pints (850 ml) water for a minimum of 3 hours. (If it's easier to soak them overnight, do so, but put them in the refrigerator to prevent fermentation.) Discard the soaking water. Add 1 pint (570 ml) fresh water to the soaked beans and bring to the boil. Reduce heat to a low simmer and cook the beans, covered, for 1 ½ hours, or until they are soft. Drain them, and set aside.

While the beans are cooking, prepare the rice. Rinse the rice to remove any foreign particles. Put it in a pot with 26 fl. oz (740 ml) water. Bring just to the boil, stir the rice once, cover, then reduce the heat to a low simmer. Cook for 40 minutes. Try not to lift the lid of the pot, or you'll have soggy rice. Shut the heat off without peeking, and let sit until serving time.

In a large frying pan, sauté the garlic, onion and pepper in olive oil until the onion is transparent and the pepper is soft. Add the cooked beans, tomatoes, tomato purée and seasonings. Stir, and let simmer while you serve the rice. Add salt and pepper to taste. Serve beans over hot rice.

Note: Pinto beans originate from Mexico. Specialist grocers may stock them.
If you prefer to use canned beans, rinse them thoroughly to remove any added sodium or preservatives.

FRIED LIVER ITALIANO

SERVES 6 TO 8

2 eggs
4 oz (115 g) whole-grain bread crumbs
2 oz (55 g) grated Parmesan
1 tsp oregano
1 lb (455 g) beef livers, cut into thin strips or cubes
1 tbsp (15 ml) olive oil
1 lb (455 g) mozzarella, cut into thin slices

Preheat the oven to 500° F (315° C, gas mark 9). Lightly grease with olive oil a 9 × 13 × 3 in (23 × 33 × 8 cm) baking tin or casserole.

In a medium-size bowl, beat the eggs. Mix the bread crumbs, Parmesan and oregano in another medium-size bowl. Put the liver pieces in the bowl with the beaten eggs. Take several pieces of the liver out of the egg mixture, shake off any excess egg, then put the pieces into the bowl with the breading mixture. Cover the pieces with the breading, then put them on a plate. Repeat this process, breading several pieces of liver at a time, until all the liver is breaded and set on the plate.

Heat the olive oil in a large frying pan. When the oil is hot but not smoking, put in the liver and let it brown on one side for about 2 minutes. Turn the pieces and repeat on the other side for 1 to 2 minutes more, or until golden brown. Remove from pan and set aside.

Repeat procedure until all the liver pieces are cooked, adding a little more olive oil if necessary. Spread half the liver pieces over the bottom of the oiled tin. Put half the mozzarella slices over the liver. Add the remaining liver, then another layer of mozzarella.

Put the tin in the preheated oven. Bake for 10 minutes, or until the cheese has melted and is a little brown. Serve with wholewheat spaghetti.

VARIATION: Add tomato sauce and a sprinkling of more Parmesan for liver parmigiana.

TROPICAL LIVER

SERVES 4

2½ fl. oz (70 ml) pineapple juice concentrate
2 tbsp (30 ml) soya sauce
1 lb (455 g) liver, cut into ½-inch cubes

2 tsp butter
4 oz (115 g) chopped spring onions
4 oz (115 g) chopped walnuts
1 lb (455 g) cooked brown rice
4 oz (115 g) chopped fresh or unsweetened canned pineapple chunks, juice reserved

Preheat the grill.

Mix the pineapple juice concentrate and soya sauce in a bowl and add the liver cubes. Set aside.

Melt the butter in a large frying pan. Add the chopped spring onions and walnuts. Sauté over low heat until the spring onions are soft. Add the rice and chopped pineapple, and sauté for 2 minutes.

Place the liver pieces in preheated grill pan. Grill for 10 minutes, turning twice; brush with the pineapple/soya marinade occasionally. When the liver is done, add it to the rice mixture. Stir until all ingredients are thoroughly combined.

Stir some of the reserved pineapple juice into the remaining marinade to make a sauce. Add it to the liver mixture as you wish, or serve separately. (Extra soy sauce can also be added, if necessary, for flavour.)

CHINESE STIR-FRY

This recipe is delicious by itself, or served over brown rice.
SERVES 4

3 tbsp (30 ml) unrefined sesame oil
1 oz (30 g) chopped spring onions
2 tsp finely chopped fresh root ginger
8 oz (225 g) hard tofu, chopped, or 8 oz (225 g) sliced meat or chicken
1 medium carrot, sliced into pieces 1/4 in (0.6 cm) thick
4 oz (115 g) sliced broccoli stems
2 oz (55 g) water chestnuts, sliced in half
8 oz (225 g) broccoli florets
4 oz (115 g) mange-tout, cut in half
3 oz (85 g) mung bean sprouts
1–1 1/2 tsp (5–7.5 ml) soya sauce
1 tbsp sesame seeds

Heat the sesame oil in a large frying pan or wok until the oil is quite warm but not hot enough to smoke or sputter. Add the chopped spring onions, and sauté till they are soft, about 5 minutes.

Add the root ginger, tofu and carrot slices. Sauté until the tofu is lightly browned, about 10 minutes. (If you are using meat, you'll need to add it later; otherwise it will be overcooked and tough.)

Push the tofu and carrots to the side of the pan.

Add the broccoli stems and water chestnuts (and meat slices if used), and sauté for 2 minutes; then add the broccoli florets and mange-tout. Sauté for 2 more minutes, then add the bean sprouts and sauté for another 2 minutes.

Add soya sauce to taste, and sprinkle with sesame seeds.

SEAFOOD RATATOUILLE

Fish can be canned tuna or mackerel that is drained and flaked, or fresh or frozen fillets, such as cod, sole or flounder. If you use frozen, try to get *deboned* fish. Otherwise, try to remove the bones as best you can. If you are using canned fish such as tuna, use three 8-oz (225-g) cans of fish packed in brine; drain them well. Scallops, although not as good nutritionally, are also quite tasty with this recipe; however, they can be prohibitively expensive.
SERVES 4

1/4 tsp oregano
1/2 tsp basil
1/4 tsp thyme
1/2 tsp rosemary
freshly ground pepper
1 medium aubergine, peeled and chopped into 1-in (2.5-cm) cubes
2 garlic cloves, minced
6 oz (170 g) courgettes, sliced
5 oz (140 g) chopped onion
1 lb (455 g) fillets of cod, sole or flounder
3 large tomatoes, diced
1 green pepper, seeded and diced
Lemon juice to taste
2 oz (55 g) chopped parsley

Preheat the oven to 375° F (190° C, gas mark 5).

Mix the herbs and pepper together in a small bowl.

Spread the aubergine cubes over the bottom of an 8 × 13 × 3 in (20 × 33 × 7.5 cm) ovenproof pan. Sprinkle half of the minced garlic over the aubergine. Sprinkle half of the herbs and pepper over, then put on a layer of all the courgette slices, followed by a layer of all the chopped onion. Bake for 15 minutes.

Cut the fillets into 1-in (2.5-cm) pieces, and set aside.

Remove the aubergine, courgette and onion mixture from the oven, and place the fish pieces in a layer on top. Sprinkle over the remaining garlic and herb mixture. Add the diced tomatoes and green pepper. Return the pan to the oven and bake another 10 minutes, or until the fish is cooked through. Remove, squeeze lemon juice on top, sprinkle with parsley and serve.

BOUILLABAISSE

My son Jeff makes this family favourite for us. Any leftover bouillabaisse can be refrigerated for up to three days and reheated for a quick meal.
SERVES 6

7 oz (200 g) chopped onions
2 garlic cloves, minced
2 large carrots, sliced
2 tbsp (30 ml) olive oil
1 lb (455 g) cod, haddock or mackerel fillets, cut into 1-in (2.5-cm) pieces
2 large tomatoes, coarsely chopped
1/2 tsp thyme
1 tsp rosemary
pinch of saffron
2 large potatoes, diced
8 fl. oz (230 ml) water
1 bay leaf
pepper to taste
1 lb (455 g) mixed uncooked oysters, scallops, prawns and mussels, as desired
1–2 oz (30–55 g) parsley sprigs

In a large pot, sauté the chopped onions, minced garlic and sliced carrots in olive oil, until the onions are transparent. Add fish, tomatoes, thyme, rosemary and saffron, and sauté for 5 minutes. Add the potatoes, water and bay leaf. Bring to the boil, reduce heat and cook for 15 minutes. Season to taste with pepper, and remove the bay leaf. Add the shellfish, cook another 5 minutes, until the prawns turn pink.

Sprinkle in parsley sprigs just before serving for a dash of colour. Serve with wholewheat bread cut into thick slices.

OVEN 'FRIED' FISH

SERVES 4 TO 5

4 fl. oz (115 ml) milk, or 1 egg, beaten
¼ tsp tarragon
2 oz (55 g) wholewheat bread crumbs
½ tsp paprika
½–1 tsp grated Parmesan
¼ tsp dry mustard
1½ lb (680 g) fish fillets
lemon juice to taste
lemon slices
sprigs of parsley

Preheat the oven to 475° F (245° C, gas mark 8). Lightly oil a baking sheet or shallow baking dish large enough to hold the fillets side by side.

In a bowl large enough to dip the fillets, place the milk or egg, add the tarragon, and combine.

In another bowl large enough to dip the fillets, mix the bread crumbs, paprika, Parmesan and mustard.

Dip each fillet into the liquid mixture, then roll it in the seasoned bread crumbs. Place the fillets on the baking sheet or in the baking dish. Bake for 7 to 10 minutes, until the fillets turn golden brown and are just done. Squeeze fresh lemon juice on top. Garnish with slices of lemon and sprigs of parsley.

Serve with brown rice and steamed vegetables. If a spread is desired, use the Basic Tofu Spread or Tomato Sauce (see recipes below).

POWER PASTA

PASTA PRIMAVERA

This keeps well for two days. Simply put any leftovers in a steamer to warm.
SERVES 6

3 tbsp (45 ml) olive oil
2 garlic cloves, minced (optional)
12 oz (340 g) sliced courgettes
8 oz (225 g) broccoli florets
4 oz (115 g) asparagus pieces, ½ in (1.2 cm) long
10 oz (285 g) carrots, cut into julienne strips

4 oz (115 g) fresh or frozen petits pois
8 oz (225 g) linguini or spaghetti
12 oz (340 g) chopped tomatoes
2 tbsp chopped fresh basil, or 1 tbsp dried

GARNISHES (optional):
Olive oil
Feta cheese
Grated Parmesan
Tomato Sauce (see recipe)
Oil and vinegar dressing
Freshly ground pepper
Minced garlic

Heat 2 tbsp (30 ml) olive oil in a large frying pan or pot. If desired, sauté minced cloves of garlic. Sauté the courgettes, broccoli, asparagus, carrots and petits pois until they are slightly soft but still crunchy, about 10 minutes.

Break the pasta into thirds. In a large pot of boiling water, place the remaining olive oil, and cook the pasta until it is *al dente*.

Drain the cooked pasta and add it to the vegetables. Mix in the tomatoes and basil, and any garnishes you wish. Stir until everything is well mixed and the flavours are blended. Serve hot.

WALNUT PESTO PASTA

SERVES 4

2 oz (55 g) walnuts
6 oz (170 g) fresh basil leaves
1 oz (30 g) chopped fresh parsley
2 garlic cloves, minced
2 oz (55 g) grated Parmesan
4–5 fl. oz (115–145 ml) olive oil
1 lb (455 g) spinach fettuccine
1 tbsp (15 ml) olive oil

Grind the walnuts in an electric blender. You may want to leave a few chunks to add a nice texture to the pesto. Add the basil, parsley, garlic, Parmesan and 4 fl. oz (115 ml) of olive oil to the walnuts. If necessary, add more olive oil until you have a thick, grainy paste.

In a large pot of boiling water to which you've added 1 tbsp (15 ml) olive oil, cook the pasta until it is *al dente*. Drain the cooked pasta, stir in the pesto and mix well.

TOFU–RICOTTA LASAGNA

SERVES 10 TO 12
TIME SAVERS: Use 24 fl. oz (680 ml) commercial tomato sauce. Be sure it
has no added sodium, sugar or preservatives. You can usually find a good
sauce in the healthfood shop. You can also use frozen spinach.

tomato sauce (see above and method)
FOR THE TOFU–RICOTTA FILLING
1 lb (455 g) firm tofu
1 lb (455 g) semi-skimmed ricotta
1 egg
2 oz (55 g) grated Parmesan
¼ tsp nutmeg
2 oz (55 g) chopped parsley

FOR THE VEGETABLE LAYER
1 lb (455 g) sliced mushrooms
2 tsp (10 ml) olive oil
*1 lb (455 g) fresh spinach, washed well, drained and chopped, or one 10-oz
    (280-g) packet frozen*

TO FINISH
9 wholewheat lasagna noodles
olive oil
12 oz (340 g) shredded semi-skimmed mozzarella
1 oz (30 g) grated Parmesan

Make the Tomato Sauce according to the directions on page 219.

TO MAKE THE TOFU–RICOTTA FILLING: Put all the ingredients in an
electric blender or food processer, and blend till you have a smooth purée.

TO MAKE THE VEGETABLE LAYER: In a large frying pan, sauté the sliced
mushrooms in the olive oil. When the mushrooms are lightly brown, add the
spinach and sauté just enough to cook slightly. If necessary, drain the
vegetable mixture.

In a large pot of boiling water to which 1 tbsp (15 ml) of olive oil has been
added, cook the lasagna until they are nearly *al dente*. Drain them and sprinkle
a little olive oil on them to prevent them from sticking together.
    Preheat the oven to 400° F (205° C, gas mark 6).

TO ASSEMBLE THE LASAGNA: Lightly oil a 9 × 13 × 2½ in (23 × 33 × 6 cm) baking dish. Spread several spoonfuls of tomato sauce on to the bottom of the dish, to keep the lasagna from sticking. Lay in 3 lasagna lengthwise, top with one-quarter of the shredded mozzarella, one-half of the vegetable mixture, one-half of the tofu–ricotta filling and about one-half of the tomato sauce. Top with 3 lasagna, then add another quarter of the shredded mozzarella, the rest of the vegetable mixture, the rest of the tofu–ricotta filling, and finish with the last 3 lasagna. Spread the remaining tomato sauce on top, then add the remaining shredded mozzarella and the grated Parmesan, mixed together.

Bake for 25 to 30 minutes, or until the cheese is lightly browned. Let stand 15 minutes before cutting, and serve hot.

CHILD-PLEASING SALADS

QUICK AND EASY PASTA SALAD

Pastas come in many interesting shapes: penne is a hollow tube with the end cut on the diagonal; rotelle or fusilli are corkscrew-shaped, and so on. It's fun to mix the different shapes, which can be appealing to children.
SERVES 4

8 oz (225 g) wholewheat pasta
olive oil to taste
12 oz (340 g) chopped tomatoes
4 oz (115 g) chopped fresh basil
black pepper and sea salt to taste

In a large pot of boiling water to which 1 tbsp (15 ml) of olive oil has been added, cook the pasta until it is *al dente*. Drain it in a colander, and run it under cold water to cool; then put in a large salad bowl. Add the tomatoes and basil. Sprinkle with olive oil. Stir. Add freshly ground black pepper and sea salt to taste.

VARIATION: For more protein, add 4 oz (115 g) chopped mozzarella.

WHITE BEAN SALAD

SERVES 6

6 oz (170 g) uncooked haricot beans
1 large bunch spinach, washed and chopped
¼ onion, sliced
2 oz (55 g) chopped walnuts
Tarragon Dressing (see p. 218)

Soak the beans in 1 pint (570 ml) hot water for a minimum of 3 hours. Discard the soak water. Put the beans in a pot with 16 fl. oz (460 ml) water, and bring just to a boil. Lower heat and simmer for 45 minutes, or until the beans are soft enough to eat, but not so that they fall apart.

Put the chopped spinach and enough water to cover it in a pot large enough to hold it, and turn on the heat. Stir the spinach constantly for 1 minute, until all pieces are slightly soft, but not wilted. Drain.

Put the cooked beans, spinach, onion and walnuts in a large salad bowl. Toss. Add tarragon dressing to taste.

SUPERIOR SOUPS

HARICOT BEAN SOUP

SERVES 4

8 oz (225 g) uncooked haricot beans
4 oz (115 g) chopped onion
2 garlic cloves, crushed
1½ tsp (7.5 ml) olive oil
2 medium carrots, chopped
2 stalks celery, chopped
¼ tsp rosemary
¼ tsp thyme
pepper and salt to taste

Rinse the beans; soak them in 1¼ pints (710 ml) of water for a minimum of 3 hours or overnight. Drain, and put them in a large heavy pot. Add 2½ pints (1.4 l) of water, bring to a boil, lower heat, and simmer, covered, until soft (about 1 hour). (If you like, replace the cooking water after 30 minutes with an equal amount of fresh water. This helps reduce the flatulence-inducing effect of the beans.)

Sauté the onion and garlic in the olive oil until soft. When the beans are cooked or nearly cooked, add the onion, garlic, carrots, celery, rosemary and thyme. Simmer another 10 minutes.

Add pepper and salt to taste.

VARIATION: Add chopped tomatoes and/or tomato purée.

QUICK AND DELICIOUS SPLIT PEA SOUP

8 oz (225 g) split peas
1¼ pints (710 ml) water
4 oz (115 g) chopped onion
4 oz (115 g) chopped celery
5 oz (140 g) sliced carrots

Wash the split peas. Put the water, split peas, onion and celery in a medium-size pot, bring just to the boil, then turn down the heat. Cover, and simmer over low heat for 40 minutes. Put the soup in a blender and purée till smooth. Then add the sliced carrots and blend briefly, just enough to have bits of carrot in the soup (unless you like it totally smooth). Return the soup to the pot and cook for another 10 minutes. Serve hot.

TASTY SPREADS, DRESSINGS, SAUCES AND DIPS

BASIC TOFU SPREAD

8 oz (225 g) silken or soft tofu
2 tbsp (30 ml) lemon juice or vinegar
¼ tsp dry mustard
⅛ tsp minced garlic, or to taste
2 tbsp (30 ml) linseed or walnut oil, or 1 tbsp (15 ml) linseed or walnut oil and 1 tbsp (15 ml) olive oil

Put the ingredients in an electric blender or food processor and blend until you have a smooth purée.

VARIATION: Add 1 tsp of herbs such as chives, dill or parsley. (This version is good as a topping for baked potatoes.)

TOFU MAYONNAISE

Tofu makes this a high-protein, high-EFA spread that you can feel good about feeding to your children. It is also easier to make than a mayonnaise with eggs. However, if you expect it to taste like egg mayonnaise, you'll be disappointed. It has its own delicate flavour.

2 tbsp (30 ml) water
1/8 tsp (0.6 ml) soya sauce
1/2 tsp (2.5 ml) apple juice concentrate
Basic Tofu Spread

Add water, soya sauce and concentrate to the Basic Tofu Spread and mix well.

TOFU SALAD DRESSING

Basic Tofu Spread
2 fl. oz (55 ml) white or tarragon vinegar
4 fl. oz (115 ml) olive oil
2 fl. oz (55 ml) linseed or walnut oil
2 tbsp (30 ml) water
1 tsp tarragon, dill or parsley

Blend the ingredients together in an electric blender or food processer. For greater tartness, use more vinegar. To make a tarragon dressing, use tarragon vinegar.

NUT BUTTER SPREADS

Smooth nut butters are a little difficult to make unless you have a hand grinder, which works best. However, you can produce a fairly successful nut butter with an electric blender. To make a nut butter, simply grind nuts or seeds in a blender or hand grinder until you have a powder, then gradually add oil until you have a paste.

If you like a chunky nut butter, simply grind for less time. A coarser grind is also less likely to produce oil separation in the nut butter.

If you use a blender, grind 4 oz (115 g) of nuts or seeds at a time. If you grind too many at once, you'll put too much stress on the blender's motor, and you won't get a fine powder.

For oils, use olive, linseed and walnut. The amount of oil depends on the type of grinder you have. A good grinder will require less oil; 1 tbsp (15 ml) oil per 4 oz (115 g) of nut or seed meal is usually enough, although you'll probably need more if you use an electric blender. The instructions that follow use an electric blender.

WALNUT BUTTER

6½ oz (185 g) walnuts
1 tbsp (15 ml) linseed oil
1 tbsp (15 ml) walnut oil
(or 2 tbsp/30 ml walnut oil alone)
1 tbsp (15 ml) water

ALMOND BUTTER

10 oz (285 g) almonds
1 tbsp (15 ml) linseed oil
2 tbsp (30 ml) walnut or olive oil
(or 3 tbsp (45 ml) walnut oil alone)
2 fl. oz (55 ml) water

SUNFLOWER BUTTER

10 oz (285 g) sunflower seeds
1 tbsp soya powder
1 tbsp (15 ml) linseed or walnut oil
1 tbsp (15 ml) tahini
2 tbsp (30 ml) water

VARIATION: To make nut butters more flavourful, add apple spread, chopped dates or raisins for sweetness. For taste, texture and additional vitamins, mix with shredded carrots, alfalfa sprouts or chopped green pepper.

Note: Keep all nut butters in the refrigerator to prevent them from becoming rancid and the oil from separating.

QUICK SANDWICH SPREAD

PREPARATION TIME: 2 minutes

4 fl. oz (115 ml) plain yoghurt
4 fl. oz (115 ml) tahini

Mix the two ingredients together in a small bowl or glass jar. Store in the refrigerator; it will keep for several days.

BASIC EGG MAYONNAISE

Be sure that all ingredients are room temperature before starting. If the oil is cold, warm it to tepid (about 70° F/21° C).

1 egg
3/4 tsp dry mustard
1 tbsp (15 ml) cider or brown rice vinegar, or lemon juice
1 tbsp (15 ml) lemon juice
8 fl. oz (230 ml) olive oil
8 fl. oz (230 ml) linseed or walnut oil

Put the egg, mustard, vinegar, and lemon juice in an electric blender. Mix the oils together in a bowl or a large measuring cup that pours easily. Blend the egg mixture; while the blender is running on a low speed, very slowly pour in the oil mixture in a thin, steady stream. Eventually the mixture will emulsify. Continue adding oil until correct consistency is obtained. (If the mayonnaise separates, remove it from the blender jar, blend another egg in the jar, then slowly pour the mayonnaise back into the jar and blend until correct consistency is obtained.)

Store in the refrigerator in a glass container.

VARIATION: For a dill mayonnaise that is delicious with cold salmon or bean salads, add to the basic mayonnaise 2½ tsp freshly chopped minced chives or the green part of a spring onion, and 1½ tsp dry dill, or to taste.

BASIC OIL AND VINEGAR DRESSING

This dressing is good for vegetable salads, bean salads or pasta.

2 fl. oz (55 ml) cider vinegar
½ tsp basil
1 garlic clove, minced
4 fl. oz (115 ml) olive oil
2 fl. oz (55 ml) linseed or walnut oil

Put the vinegar, basil and garlic in an electric blender. Blend briefly, then add the combined oils slowly.

VARIATION: For a tarragon dressing that is great with beans, use tarragon vinegar and 1 tsp tarragon in place of the cider vinegar and basil.

TAHINI–GINGER DRESSING

This keeps well in the refrigerator, although it may thicken. Just add more water to thin.

1 tsp minced root ginger
1 tsp finely minced spring onion
2–3 tbsp (30–45 ml) lemon juice
1 tsp (5 ml) soya sauce
4 fl. oz (115 ml) tahini
2½ fl. oz (70 ml) water

Place all the ingredients in a blender, adding the water last as needed, and purée until well incorporated.

TOMATO SAUCE

TIME SAVER: Prepare ahead, then freeze.

2 lb (910 g) plum tomatoes, peeled and chopped
1 medium onion, chopped
3 garlic cloves, minced
1 tbsp (15 ml) olive oil
2 tsp dried basil
½–1 tsp dried oregano
½ tsp thyme
6 oz (170 g) tomato purée
3 tbsp cooked lentils (optional)

Put the plum tomatoes in a blender or food processer and process to a coarse mixture. In a large heavy pot, sauté the onion and garlic in the olive oil until soft. Add the tomatoes, herbs and tomato purée, and stir well to combine thoroughly.

For a meatier flavour and a heartier sauce, with more minerals and protein, add the lentils.

Simmer over low heat, uncovered, for at least 30 minutes, stirring occasionally. The longer it cooks, the better it will be.

HUMMUS

TIME SAVERS: If you can't face the thought of cooking the chickpeas from scratch, use canned ones. However, purchase those with no added salt or preservatives. If the only brands in your market contain added sodium, rinse them very well (at least 3 times) to wash off as much of the additives as possible.

8 oz (225 g) chickpeas
2½ fl. oz (70 ml) lemon juice
2 garlic cloves, minced
2½ fl. oz (70 ml) tahini
2 tbsp (30 ml) linseed or walnut oil
¼ tsp chilli powder

Soak chickpeas in 1½ pints (850 ml) water for 4 hours, or overnight. Discard the water. Bring 2 pints (1.1 l) of fresh water to a boil, add the soaked chickpeas, cover and simmer over low heat for 2 hours, or until soft and easily mashed with a fork. (To help reduce the 'wind'-inducing effect of the chickpeas, replace the cooking water with an equal amount of fresh water after 1 hour of cooking.) Drain the chickpeas, reserving the stock.

Put cooked chickpeas in an electric blender or food processer, add the lemon juice, garlic, tahini, linseed oil, and chilli powder. Blend slowly, using chickpea stock as necessary to obtain the desired consistency. Chill. Use as a sandwich spread or dip.

MEXICAN BEAN DIP

1 oz (30 g) chopped onion
1 garlic clove, minced
2 tbsp finely chopped celery
1 tbsp (15 ml) olive oil
12 oz (340 g) cooked kidney or pinto beans (see p. 205)
¼ tsp (1.25 ml) soya sauce
ground cumin and cayenne to taste

Sauté the onion, garlic and celery in the olive oil. Add the beans and seasonings, and stir until well mixed. Put the ingredients in a blender or food processer and purée until smooth. Serve with warmed tortillas or wholewheat pita bread.

TOFU–CARROT–DILL DIP

This dip keep for several days if refrigerated. It will separate when it is stored; just stir before serving.

2 tbsp (30 ml) olive oil
1 tbsp (15 ml) linseed or walnut oil
2 tbsp (30 ml) lemon juice
1 tbsp (15 ml) water
1 tsp (5 ml) soya sauce
8 oz (225 g) sliced carrots
1 1/2 tbsp finely chopped spring onion, green part only
1 garlic clove, minced
1 tsp dried dillweed
6 oz (170 g) firm tofu

Place everything except the tofu in a blender or food processer and blend briefly, until carrots are coarsely chopped. Add tofu, blend well, until a fairly grainy texture is achieved. Serve with raw vegetables and pita bread.

NUTRIENT-DENSE SNACKS AND SWEETS

QUICK PIZZA

For a pizza crust, use either wholewheat muffins or baps or wholewheat pita bread. For the topping, use beefsteak tomatoes or plum tomatoes, shredded mozzarella cheese, grated Parmesan, dried oregano, dried or fresh basil, minced garlic (optional – the children may not like it) and olive oil. If you like, add a little variety and a few more vitamins and minerals by including other vegetables, such as sliced courgettes or mushrooms.

MAKES 2 SERVINGS PER WHOLE-GRAIN MUFFIN/BAP, OR 4 SERVINGS PER WHOLEWHEAT PITA.

FOR A MUFFIN OR BAP

2 slices beefsteak tomato, or 1/2 plum tomato, chopped
3 oz (85 g) shredded mozzarella
1 tsp grated Parmesan
1/8 tsp dried oregano and 1/8 tsp basil, mixed together
1/4 tsp (1.25 ml) olive oil

FOR A PITA BREAD
3 plum tomatoes, chopped
½ medium courgette, sliced into thin discs
2 large mushrooms, thinly sliced
4 oz (115 g) shredded mozzarella
1 tbsp grated Parmesan
¼ tsp dried oregano
¼ tsp dried basil
½ tsp minced garlic
1 tsp (5 ml) olive oil

Preheat the oven to 425° F (220° C, gas mark 6).

Split the muffin or pita bread in half and put the halves on a baking sheet. (If you like a dry crust, lightly toast the bread in a toaster or oven before adding the toppings.)

Divide ingredients evenly between muffin halves or pita halves, reserving the olive oil. Drizzle the olive oil on top.

Bake for 10 to 15 minutes, or until the cheese is melted and the tomato is soft. Let cool for 5 minutes before serving.

FRUIT SORBET

BASIC INGREDIENTS

2 oz (55 g) powdered milk or 1 packet unflavoured gelatine, dissolved in 5 fl. oz (140 ml) warm orange, apple or pineapple juice (see Note)
6 oz (170 g) fruit juice concentrate, such as apple or orange
3 medium ripe bananas, or ¾ lb (340 g) fresh or frozen blueberries, blackcurrants or blackberries, or 1 lb (455 g) crushed fresh or canned pineapple (see Note), or ½ lb (225 g) fresh or frozen strawberries

BASIC PROCEDURE: Mix the powdered milk or gelatine dissolved in fruit juice with the fruit juice concentrate in a blender or food processor. (For a creamier sorbet, increase the amount of powdered milk.) Add 2 or 3 fruits, as preferred, and blend again for 5 minutes, or until smooth.

Pour into ice cube trays or moulds and freeze until firm. If moulds are not available, use small paper cups (2½ fl. oz/70 ml capacity). Put an ice lolly stick (available in some supermarkets or variety stores) in the centre.

Note: It is preferable nutritionally to have milk in the sorbet. If a dairy-free sorbet is desired, use the gelatine dissolved in warm fruit juice. Canned pineapple should appear in the sorbet on its own.

BANANA–STRAWBERRY SORBET

*5 fl. oz (140 ml) fresh orange juice, or 4 fl. oz (115 ml) water plus 2 tbsp (30
   ml) orange juice concentrate
1 packet unflavoured gelatine
6 oz (170 g) frozen orange juice concentrate
3 medium bananas
5 oz (140 g) hulled fresh strawberries, washed*

Put the orange juice or water and orange juice mixture in the blender. Add all
the other ingredients, and blend until you have a smooth purée. Pour this
mixture into 2 ice cube trays or 10 moulds. (If moulds are used, place ice lolly
sticks in the centre.) Freeze several hours or overnight, until firm.

   To serve, blend the frozen sorbet cubes to make a smooth mixture. Serve,
decorated with a sprig of fresh mint and/or a fresh strawberry. Ice lollies are
removed from moulds and eaten off the stick.

PINEAPPLE–BANANA SORBET

*5 fl. oz (140 ml) water
5 fl. oz (140 ml) orange juice concentrate
3 medium bananas
1 lb (455 g) pineapple, cubed*

Follow the same directions as for Banana–Strawberry Sorbet.

BLACKCURRANT–APPLE SORBET

*2 oz (55 g) powdered milk
5 fl. oz (140 ml) apple juice, or 4 fl. oz (115 ml) water plus 2 tbsp (30 ml) apple
   juice concentrate
6 oz (170 g) apple juice concentrate
3 medium bananas
12 oz (340 g) fresh blackcurrants*

Follow the directions in the master recipe.

YOGHURT ICE LOLLIES

*8–10 oz (225–280 g) frozen orange juice concentrate, or 2 lb (910 g) fresh
   strawberries or one 20-oz (565-g) pkg frozen
16 fl. oz (460 ml) plain yoghurt or soft or silken tofu*

If you use strawberries, purée the fresh or frozen berries in a blender. Then add them (or the orange juice if you are using that instead) to the yoghurt or tofu and blend again. Transfer to moulds and freeze for several hours or overnight, until firm. Insert ice lolly sticks for handles when lollies are semi-firm. Unmould to serve.

YOGHURT–STRAWBERRY ICE LOLLIES

1 lb (455 g) fresh strawberries
8 fl. oz (230 ml) plain yoghurt
2 fl. oz (55 ml) apple juice concentrate (optional)

Prepare as instructed in master recipe, using apple juice concentrate if purée isn't sweet enough.

FRUIT ICE

Blend fresh fruit – strawberries, pineapple or watermelon. Freeze in an ice cube tray, then blend again until smooth. Serve in small dishes, or refreeze in small paper cups.

You can also use frozen fruit: a 20-oz (565 g) package of frozen strawberries will yield 16 fl. oz (460 ml) purée.

BANANA ICE

Peel a banana and cut into chunks. Put the chunks on greaseproof paper and freeze until hard. Put the frozen chunks in a blender and blend until you have a smooth, creamy consistency. Occasionally stop the blender and stir the chunks with a rubber spatula to facilitate blending. If you have a difficult time, add ½ to 1 unfrozen banana or some milk or yoghurt.

For a little variation, add vanilla extract and/or other frozen fruits. A favourite is a mixture of strawberries and banana.

It's fun to make banana splits with the children. Put slices of unfrozen banana in a small bowl. Add different kinds of homemade fruit ices and banana ice. Pour a little orange or pineaple juice concentrate over the top, then sprinkle with desiccated coconut, chopped nuts and seeds and raisins.

RICE PUDDING

This is a delicious rice pudding that isn't sweet.
SERVES 6

2 oz (55 g) long-grain brown rice
14 fl. oz (400 ml) water
3 oz (85 g) raisins
4 eggs
24 fl. oz (680 ml) low-fat milk
2 tsp (10 ml) vanilla extract
½ tsp ground cinnamon, or ¼ tsp grated nutmeg (see Note)

Rinse the brown rice, cleaning it well. Put it and water in a pot. Bring the water just to the boil, cover and turn the heat down very low. Simmer for 50 minutes. The rice should be a little wetter than usual.

Preheat the oven to 350° F (175° C, gas mark 4).

Put the raisins in a small bowl and add hot water to cover plus 1 in (2.5 cm). Let the raisins plump for 10 minutes. Lightly beat the eggs, add the milk and vanilla, and cinnamon, if desired. Lightly butter a 3 pint (1.7 l) baking dish.

When the rice is cooked, add it to the liquid mixture and stir, mixing well. Drain the raisins. Stir them into the rice mixture.

Pour the pudding into the buttered baking dish. Bake for 35 to 40 minutes, or until the pudding is set. (It is set when a knife inserted into the side comes out clean. The centre may seem too wet still. Don't worry, it will continue to cook and set after you take it out of the oven. Overcooking will cause it to collapse and turn to liquid.)

Sprinkle the top with cinnamon or nutmeg if you haven't added it yet. Let sit a few minutes before serving. Or serve cold.

Note: If you love the taste of cinnamon, add it to the pudding rather than sprinkling it on top.

TOFU CUSTARD

A high-protein, mineral-rich, delicious pudding.
SERVES 4

3 eggs
8 fl. oz (230 ml) firm tofu
2 tbsp (30 ml) rice malt sweetener, or 2 fl. oz (55 ml) honey
8 fl. oz (230 ml) milk

1 tsp (5 ml) vanilla extract
½ tsp ground cinnamon
⅛ tsp nutmeg (optional)

Preheat the oven to 350° F (175° C, gas mark 4). Lightly butter a 2½ pint (1.4 l) casserole dish.

Beat the eggs in a medium-size bowl. In a blender or food processer, blend the tofu, sweetener or honey, milk, vanilla and cinnamon until smooth. Pour the blended mixture into the bowl with the beaten eggs, and stir, mixing well.

Pour the custard mixture into the buttered casserole dish. Bake for 1 hour. Sprinkle with nutmeg before serving, if desired.

TOFU–ORANGE PUDDING

SERVES 6

16 fl. oz (460 ml) silken tofu
2 small bananas
4 fl. oz (115 ml) orange juice concentrate
2 tsp (10 ml) vanilla extract
4 fl. oz (115 ml) buttermilk
grated orange peel (optional)
sprig of mint (optional)
chopped nuts (optional)

Put all the ingredients except optional garnishes in a blender or food processer. Blend until smooth. Pour into individual serving dishes (glass-stemmed dessert dishes look nice). Chill about 1 hour, until a nice pudding texture is achieved.

If you wish, decorate with grated orange peel and a sprig of mint, or sprinkle chopped nuts on top.

AMBROSIA

SERVES 6

4 oranges, peeled and sliced
3 oz (85 g) unsweetened desiccated coconut
1 tbsp (15 ml) orange juice concentrate
2½ fl. oz (70 ml) pineapple juice, or 1 tbsp (15 ml) pineapple juice concentrate
*   mixed with 2 fl. oz (55 ml) water*
whole strawberry (optional)
chopped walnuts, sliced almonds or sesame seeds (optional)

Put the orange slices in a large bowl. Add the coconut and mix thoroughly. In a separate bowl, mix the orange juice concentrate and pineapple juice or pineapple juice concentrate and water. Pour this mixture over the orange slices and coconut. Stir again.

Refrigerate for 1 hour before serving. Put the ambrosia in glass dessert dishes. Top with a whole strawberry, or sprinkle with chopped walnuts, sliced almonds or sesame seeds.

PEANUT BUTTER CHEWS

These are fun to make with children. 'Little hands' can help you blend the dough by kneading it.

MAKES 24 CHEWS

6 oz (170 g) rolled oats
2 oz (55 g) sunflower seeds
4 oz (115 g) raisins (see Note)
4 fl. oz (115 ml) peanut butter
4 fl. oz (115 ml) apple juice concentrate

Preheat the oven to 350° F (175° C, gas mark 4).

Put the rolled oat, sunflower seeds and raisins into a large mixing bowl. Mix, then add other ingredients and mix well until combined. Let the mixture sit a minute so that the oats can soak up some of the moisture. Meanwhile, lightly oil a baking sheet.

Shape the dough into tablespoon-size pieces, and put them on the baking sheet. Flatten them slightly.

Bake for 12 minutes, or until lightly browned. Let cool on a wire rack.

Store in an airtight container in the refrigerator. They keep for several days.

Note: If the raisins are too dry or hard, soak them in hot water a few minutes to allow them to plump; then drain and use.

SESAME–SPICE OATMEAL BISCUITS

It takes lots less time if you have small helping hands to form these biscuits. Making oatmeal biscuits is a great opportunity for fun in the kitchen with your children.

MAKES 100 BISCUITS

8 oz (225 g) pitted dates

8 fl. oz (230 ml) orange juice, or 2 fl. oz (55 ml) orange juice concentrate plus 6
　fl. oz (170 ml) water
2 oz (55 g) butter, melted
12 oz (340 g) rolled oats
4 oz (115 g) wholewheat flour
½ tsp baking soda
½ tsp ground cinnamon
pinch of ground cloves
pinch of grated nutmeg
pinch of ground ginger
8 oz (225 g) raisins
4 oz (115 g) sesame seeds
4 fl. oz (115 ml) linseed or walnut oil

Preheat the oven to 350° F (175° C, gas mark 4). Lightly oil two baking sheets. Place pitted dates in a medium-size saucepan, and cover with the orange juice or orange juice concentrate and water. Simmer until soft.

In a large bowl, combine the rolled oats, flour, baking soda and spices. Add the raisins and sesame seeds to the dry mixture, stirring so that the raisins are covered with flour.

By now the dates should be soft. Put the dates and their liquid, the melted butter and linseed or walnut oil in a blender or food processer. Purée until smooth. Pour this mixture into the dry ingredients. Stir until well mixed.

Drop the dough by heaping teaspoonfuls on to the oiled baking sheets. Bake for 15 minutes, or until biscuits are brown around the edges. Cool on a rack.

BANANA–NUT OATMEAL BISCUITS

MAKES 24 BISCUITS

8 oz (225 g) rolled oats
3 oz (85 g) chopped walnuts, pecans or sunflower seeds
8 oz (225 g) raisins
3 medium bananas
1½ oz (40 g) butter, melted
2½ tbsp (35 ml) linseed or walnut oil
1 tsp (5 ml) orange juice concentrate

Preheat the oven to 350° F (175° C, gas mark 4). Lightly butter and flour a baking sheet. In a large bowl, combine the rolled oats, nuts and raisins.

Put the bananas, melted butter, oil and orange juice concentrate in a blender or food processor, and blend until you have a smooth liquid.

Add the liquid mixture to the oat mixture and mix well, until the oats have absorbed the liquid and are fairly soft.

Drop the dough by tablespoonfuls on to the buttered and floured baking sheet, leaving ½ inch (1.2 cm) between the biscuits. They do not spread as they bake, so shape them as you wish them to look. Bake for 20 to 25 minutes, or until brown around the edges. Cool on a rack.

DATE–NUT BARS

These are a chewy sandwich biscuit, with a delicious date filling.
MAKES 36 1½ IN (3.7 CM) SQUARE BARS

FOR THE FILLING
8 oz (225 g) pitted dates
4 fl. oz (115 ml) orange juice concentrate
3 oz (85 g) chopped walnuts

FOR THE CRUST
6 oz (170 g) wholewheat flour
5 oz (140 g) rolled oats
1 oz (30 g) nuts or seeds, (e.g. almonds, sunflower, flaxseed, walnuts), ground
1 tsp baking soda
1 tsp ground cinnamon
1 egg
4 fl. oz (115 ml) buttermilk
6 oz (170 g) orange juice concentrate

Preheat the oven to 400° F (205° C, gas mark 6). Lightly butter a 9 × 13 × 2 in (23 × 32 × 5 cm) baking pan.

TO MAKE THE FILLING: Put the filling ingredients in a medium-size saucepan over low heat, and let them soften for a few minutes. Mash the softened ingredients together until the concentrate is absorbed and you have a spreadable paste. Set aside.

TO MAKE THE CRUST: In a large bowl, combine the flour, oats, ground nuts or seeds, baking soda and cinnamon. In a small bowl, beat together the egg, buttermilk and orange juice concentrate. Add the liquid mixture to the dry ingredients. Stir the dough until well mixed.

TO ASSEMBLE THE BARS: Spread half the dough for the crust in the bottom of the lightly buttered pan, using a wet rubber spatula. You may have to moisten the spatula several times in order to spread the dough evenly.

Spread the filling mixture over the crust, also using a moistened rubber spatula. Then top with the remaining crust mixture, again spreading with a wet rubber spatula.

Bake for 30 to 35 minutes. Cut 1½-in (3.7-cm) squares with a sharp knife while the bars are warm. Remove them from the pan and let them cool on wire racks. Be careful with the filling; it will be fiery hot.

PUMPKIN BISCUITS

MAKES 60 BISCUITS

2 eggs
3 oz (85 g) apple juice concentrate
3 oz (85 g) orange juice concentrate
2 tbsp (30 ml) yoghurt
12 oz (340 g) pumpkin, either cooked fresh or canned, with no additives
10 oz (280 f) wholewheat flour
1 tsp ground cinnamon
½ tsp grated nutmeg
1 tsp baking soda
8 oz (225 g) raisins
6 oz (170 g) seeds, such as pumpkin or sunflower, or chopped nuts, such as
    walnuts

Preheat the oven to 375° F (190° C, gas mark 5), and lightly oil two baking sheets.

Put the eggs, juice concentrates, yoghurt and pumpkin in a blender, and purée well. In a large bowl, mix the remaining ingredients, then add the wet ingredients. Stir just until combined but don't overmix or the biscuits will be tough.

Drop the dough by tablespoonfuls on to the lightly oiled baking sheets. These biscuits do not spread when baked, so shape the dough as you wish – either in balls, or flattened slightly.

Bake in the preheated oven for 15 to 18 minutes, or until puffed and browned. Cool on a rack.

MUESLI BARS

Once you've made your muesli, these bars are a snap. The longer you keep them, the better they are. Two to three days after making them, they're even better than they are fresh.

MAKES 48 1¼ IN (3 CM) SQUARE BARS

3 eggs
3 tbsp (45 ml) apple juice concentrate
1 tsp ground cinnamon
enough of Muesli I (see p. 201) to equal 24 fl. oz (690 ml)
4–8 oz (115–225 g) raisins (see Note)

Preheat the oven to 350° F (175° C, gas mark 4).

In a large bowl, beat together the eggs, apple juice concentrate and cinnamon. Add the muesli and raisins, and mix well. Let the mixture sit in order to absorb some moisture while you lightly oil a 9 in (23 cm) square baking pan. Spread the mixture evenly in the pan, and pat it down with the back of a large spoon.

Bake for 25 minutes, or until set and lightly brown around the edges. While the mixture is still warm, cut into 1¼ in (3 cm) squares. Store in the refrigerator.

Note: If your muesli already contains raisins, use only 4 oz (115 g) additional; if it has no raisins, use 8 oz (225 g) raisins.

FRUIT AND NUT TREATS

MAKES ABOUT 45 ¾ IN (1.9 CM) PATTIES

about 18 pitted dates
about 8 dried figs, stems cut off
3 tbsp (45 ml) orange juice concentrate
2 tbsp (30 ml) hot water
9 oz (255 g) ground almonds and walnuts
1½ oz (45 g) ground linseed (see Note)

Put the dried fruit, orange juice concentrate and hot water in a medium-size bowl. Mash the ingredients with a potato masher or a wooden spoon, until you have a fairly smooth mixture. (A few lumps are fine.)

Combine the nuts and seeds in a small bowl. Remove the equivalent of 4 fl. oz (115 ml) of this mixture and set aside in a cup. (You will use this mixture to coat the patties.)

Add the remaining mixture to the fruit and liquid mixture, and mix well. To form the treats, take a small ball of dough and press it flat slightly to make a ¾ in (1.9 cm) pattie. Put the pattie in the cup of ground nuts and seeds and coat thoroughly.

Keep the patties in a sealed container in the refrigerator.

Note: Linseed may be ground in a coffee grinder or a nut and seed grinder.

VARIATION: If desired, ½ oz (15 g) desiccated coconut and ¼ tsp almond extract can be added to the mixture.

NUT BUTTER–COCONUT TREATS

MAKES 40 SWEETS

8 fl. oz (230 ml) peanut or walnut butter, or 6 fl. oz (170 ml) peanut butter and
  2 fl. oz (55 ml) walnut butter
6 oz (170 g) chopped raisins, dates or figs
6 oz (170 g) unsweetened desiccated coconut
3 oz (85 g) nuts and seeds (e.g. walnuts, sunflower seeds, linseed), ground

In a medium-size bowl, mix the nut butter, dried fruit and coconut. Make small balls or 1 in (2.5 cm) patties. Roll them in the ground nuts and seeds. Keep in the refrigerator.

BASIC SPICE BREAD

This dessert bread recipe is also the basis for a banana or carrot bread.
MAKES ONE 6 × 10 IN (15 × 25 CM) LOAF

6 oz (170 g) wholewheat pastry flour
2 oz (55 g) soya flour
1 tsp baking soda
2 tsp ground cinnamon
¼ tsp grated nutmeg
¼ tsp ground allspice
4 oz (115 g) raisins
3 oz (85 g) chopped walnuts
2 oz (55 g) sesame seeds
3 eggs
6 fl. oz (170 ml) plain yoghurt
2 oz (55 g) butter, melted
2 fl. oz (55 ml) linseed or walnut oil
6 fl. oz (170 ml) orange juice concentrate

Preheat the oven to 350° F (175° C, gas mark 4). Lightly butter a 6 × 10 in (15 × 25 cm) loaf pan.
  In a large bowl, sift together the flours, baking soda and spices. Then add

the raisins, walnuts and sesame seeds. Mix until they are coated with flour to prevent them from sinking to the bottom of the dough.

In another large bowl, beat the eggs, yoghurt, melted butter, oil and orange juice concentrate until they are blended. Stir the liquid ingredients into the dry, blending but not beating.

Pour into the prepared pan and bake for 40 minutes.

BANANA BREAD

Make the following changes to the Basic Spice Bread recipe:

Substitute 4 fl. oz (115 ml) orange juice concentrate for the 6 fl. oz (170 ml)
Substitute 2 fl. oz (55 ml) yoghurt for the 6 fl. oz (170 ml)
Substitute ½ tsp ground allspice for the ¼ tsp
Add 12 fl. oz (340 ml) mashed bananas (5 small or 2 to 3 medium) to the liquid ingredients

Put the liquid ingredients in a blender instead of in a small bowl and blend until smooth. Then add the moist ingredients to the flour mixture and mix as directed.

Pour into the prepared pan and bake at 350° F (175° C, gas mark 4) for 1 hour.

CARROT BREAD

Make the following changes to the Basic Spice Bread recipe:

Substitute 4 fl. oz (115 ml) orange juice concentrate for the 6 fl. oz (170 ml)
Substitute 2 fl. oz (55 ml) yoghurt for the 6 fl. oz (170 m)
Substitute ½ tsp ground allspice for the ¼ tsp
Add about 9 oz (255 g) grated carrot to the liquid ingredients

Pour the batter into the prepared pan, and bake at 350° F (175° C, gas mark 4) for 1 hour.

PUMPKIN PIE

This pie is denser than most pumpkin pies, but the texture is very good when served cold. If you prefer a lighter pie, however, add the optional egg whites.
MAKES 6 SERVINGS

FOR THE PASTRY CRUST
5 oz (140 g) wholewheat pastry flour
4 oz (115 g) cold butter

2 tbsp (30 ml) linseed or walnut oil
1 egg (optional)
cold water (optional)

FOR THE FILLING
1 lb (455 g) cooked fresh or canned pumpkin
8 oz (225 g) firm tofu
3 tbsp (45 ml) apple juice concentrate
1 tsp (5 ml) vanilla
2 tsp ground cinnamon
1/2 tsp ground allspice
4 tbsp (60 ml) honey
2 egg whites (optional)

TO MAKE THE PASTRY CRUST: Preheat the oven to 425° F (220° C, gas mark 6). Put the flour into a medium-size bowl. Cut the butter into 8 pieces, and add them to the flour. Use your fingers to blend the butter into the flour, or cut it in with a pastry blender, until it resembles coarse crumbs. Sprinkle the oil into the flour-and-butter mixture as you work. Do not overmix, or you'll have a tough crust.

For a flakier crust, beat the egg in a small bowl, then add it to the pastry mixture. Stir it in quickly and lightly with a fork.

Form the dough into a ball. If it is too dry, add a little cold water. Roll out the dough into a 10 inch (25 cm) circle on lightly floured greaseproof paper with a lightly floured rolling pin. (To prevent the greaseproof paper from slipping as you roll, sprinkle a little water under it on your work surface.)

Turn the greaseproof paper over on to a 9 in (23 cm) pie plate so that the rolled crust falls into the pie plate. Crimp the edges, and prick the bottom of the crust in several places with a fork, to prevent the crust from bubbling up when it bakes. Bake it for 8 to 10 minutes, or until it is lightly browned.

Lower the heat to 350° F (175° C, gas mark 4), then prepare the filling.

TO MAKE THE FILLING: Place all filling ingredients except the egg whites in a blender, and blend well.

If you are adding the egg whites for a lighter texture, beat them in a small bowl until stiff. Pour the filling mixture into a large bowl, then fold in the egg whites.

Pour the filling into the baked pie shell. Bake for 40 minutes. Refrigerate before serving.

SMOOTHIES

All smoothies must include the following, to provide essential nutrients: 3 tbsp (45 ml) yoghurt or tofu, 1 small banana, and 1 tbsp (15 ml) linseed or walnut oil. Note that, when using tofu, silken tofu works the best, but firm and soft tofu are also satisfactory. Blend all ingredients in a blender or food processer until you have a smooth drink. You can also freeze the mixtures in moulds to make ice lollies.

Following are five different delicious smoothies:

ALMOND–YOGHURT

10 almonds
4 fl. oz (115 ml) water
3 tbsp (45 ml) yoghurt
1 small banana
1 tbsp (15 ml) orange juice concentrate
1 tbsp (15 ml) linseed or walnut oil

Grind the almonds in the blender, then add all the remaining ingredients and liquefy.

WALNUT–ORANGE

1 oz (30 g) walnuts
1 tbsp (15 ml) orange juice concentrate
4 fl. oz (115 ml) water
1 small banana, or 5 pitted dates
1 tsp desiccated coconut
3 tbsp (45 ml) yoghurt
1 tbsp (15 ml) linseed or walnut oil

Grind the walnuts in the blender, then add all the remaining ingredients and liquefy.

TOFU–FIG

1 1/2 oz (40 g) tofu
1 small banana
4 figs
1 tbsp (15 ml) orange juice concentrate
6 fl. oz (170 ml) water

1 tbsp (15 ml) linseed or walnut oil
1 tbsp oat bran

Blend all ingredients together in a blender.

PINEAPPLE–TOFU

4 fl. oz (115 ml) pineapple juice, or 1 tbsp (15 ml) pineapple juice concentrate
    and 4 fl. oz (115 ml) water
1 egg, or 1½ oz (40 g) tofu
1 small banana
1 tbsp (15 ml) linseed or walnut oil
3 tbsp (45 ml) yoghurt
8 oz (225 g) strawberries (optional)

Blend all ingredients together in a blender.

TAHINI–BANANA

1 tbsp (15 ml) tahini
1 small banana
1½ oz (40 g) tofu
1 tbsp (15 ml) linseed or walnut oil
2 tbsp (30 ml) pineapple juice concentrate
5 fl. oz (145 ml) water

Blend all ingredients together in a blender.

GOOD-FOR-YOU ICINGS AND TOPPINGS

VANILLA TOFU ICING

The ground, soaked linseed in this icing recipe provides nutritional value and
helps hold the icing together. It will also add little brown specks to the icing. If
you cannot get or make ground linseed, just eliminate. The icing will still hold
very well without it.

**MAKES ENOUGH TO COAT THINLY TOP AND SIDES OF ONE 9 IN
(23 CM) CAKE**

6 oz (160 g) firm tofu
2 tsp ground linseed soaked in 2 tsp (10 ml) water (optional)

2 tsp (10 ml) lemon juice
3 tbsp (45 ml) apple juice concentrate
1 tsp (5 ml) vanilla extract

Put the tofu in a blender and mash lightly with a rubber spatula. Add the other ingredients and blend until you have a smooth icing. (It should be neither runny nor stiff.) Refrigerate, covered, to thicken further. It can be spread with a rubber spatula before or after refrigeration.

ORANGE TOFU ICING

6 oz (170 g) firm tofu
2 tsp ground linseed soaked in 2 tsp (10 ml) water
3 tbsp (45 ml) orange juice concentrate
1 oz (30 g) banana
grated orange peel

Follow instructions in the master recipe for preparing the icing, reserving the grated orange peel. Top iced cake or muffins with the grated orange peel for additional colour and vitamin C.

COCONUT TOFU ICING

6 oz (170 g) firm tofu
2 tsp ground linseed soaked in 2 tsp (10 ml) water
3 tbsp (45 ml) pineapple juice concentrate
1 oz (30 g) banana
3 tbsp desiccated coconut
extra coconut for topping (optional)

Follow instructions in the master recipe for preparing the icing. Top iced cake or muffins with more coconut, if you like.

PANCAKE AND WAFFLE TOPPINGS

Delicious toppings can be prepared from fresh, frozen, canned or dried fruits. If a fruit is dry or not very sweet, 2 tsp (10 ml) of fruit concentrate can be added to the mixture to sweeten and moisten it. Orange, apple or pineapple concentrates are available in supermarkets. You can use canned, crushed pineapple, but be certain it has no sugar syrup or other kinds of sweeteners. If you use frozen fruits, be sure there is no added sugar or other additives. To use frozen fruit, remove it from the freezer the night before, and let it defrost overnight in the refrigerator. Note that frozen fruits often have a different taste and consistency from fresh – blueberries, for example, are usually smaller and sometimes less tasty.

FRESH FRUIT SPREAD

Blueberries, raspberries, peaches, apricots, apples, papaya, strawberries or
  pineapple
¹/₃ banana (optional)
2 tbsp (30 ml) yoghurt (optional)
2 tbsp (30 ml) apple sauce (optional)
2 tsp desiccated coconut (optional)
¹/₄ tsp ground cinnamon (optional)
2 tsp (10 ml) fruit concentrate (optional)

Blend fresh or frozen fruit in a blender or food processer. A 8 fl. oz (230 ml) measure of fruit will yield about 4 fl. oz (115 ml) purée. If you like a chunky sauce, don't run the blender very long; if you want a thicker sauce, add the banana. Any of the remaining ingredients can be added to enhance the flavour of the spread.

Try the following variations, or devise your own.

PEACH AND BANANA
MAKES ENOUGH FOR 4 TO 6 PANCAKES

¹/₂ large banana
1 ripe peach, peeled and pitted
¹/₄ tsp ground cinnamon

Put all the ingredients in a blender, and blend until you have a smooth sauce.

CINNAMON APPLE SAUCE
MAKES ENOUGH FOR 4 TO 6 PANCAKES

¹/₄ tsp ground cinnamon
6 fl. oz (170 ml) unsweetened apple sauce

Mix the cinnamon into the apple sauce. If you like a warm topping, heat the mixture about 1 minute.

YOGHURT–TAHINI SYRUP
MAKES 5 FL. OZ (145 ML)

2 fl. oz (55 ml) tahini
2 fl. oz (55 ml) yoghurt
½ tsp ground cinnamon
1 tbsp (15 ml) water
1 tbsp (15 ml) apple juice concentrate

Stir the ingredients together in a small bowl until they are well mixed.

References

CHAPTER 1: THE VITAL LINK

1. A. S. Kozlovsky *et al.*, ' Effects of diets high in simple sugars on urinary chromium losses', *Metabolism* 35 (1986): 515–18.
2. D. Toth, 'Actual new cancer-causing hydrazines, hydrazides and hydrazones', *Journal of Cancer Research and Clinical Oncology* 97 (1980): 97–108. B. Toth & J. Erickson, 'Reversal of the toxicity of hydrazine analogues by pyridoxine hydrochloride', *Toxicology* 7 (1977): 31–6.
3. R. A. Shakman, 'Nutritional influences on the toxicity of environmental pollutants', *Archives of Environmental Health* 28 (1974): 105–13.
4. L. Galland, 'Increased requirements for essential fatty acids in atopic individuals: a review with clinical descriptions', *Journal of the American College of Nutrition* 5 (1986): 213–28.
5. M. S. Manku *et al.*, 'Reduced levels of prostaglandin precursors in the blood of atopic patients: defective delta-6-desaturate function as a biochemical basis for atopy', *Prostaglandins, Leukotrienes in Medicine* 9 (1982): 615–28, M. S. Manku *et al.*, 'Essential fatty acids in the plasma phospholipids of patients with atopic eczema', *British Journal of Dermatology* 110 (1984): 643–8.
6. R. E. Rocklin *et al.*, 'Altered arachidonic acid content in polymorphonuclear and mononuclear cells from patients with allergic rhinitis and/or asthma', *Lipids* 21 (1986): 17–20.

CHAPTER 2: PREGNANCY

1. L. Tallarigo *et al.*, 'Relation of glucose tolerance to complications of pregnancy in non-diabetic women', *New England Journal of Medicine* 315 (1987): 989–92.
2. S. Monarca *et al.*, 'Mutagenicity assessment of different drinking water supplies before and after treatments', *Bulletin of Environmental and Contamination Toxicology* 34 (1985): 815–23.
3. J. E. Blundell & A. J. Hill, 'Paradoxical effects of an intense sweetener (aspartame) on appetite', *Lancet* 1 (1986): 1092–3. S. D. Stellman & L. Garfinkel, 'Artificial sweetener use and one-year weight change among women', *Preventive Medicine* 15 (1986): 195–8.
4. M. Stjernfeldt *et al.*, 'Maternal smoking during pregnancy and risk of childhood cancer', *Lancet* 1 (1986): 1350–3.
5. C. Burchfield *et al.*, 'Passive smoking in childhood', *American Review of Respiratory Diseases* 133 (1986): 966–70. Y. Chen *et al.*, 'Influence of passive smoking on admissions for respiratory illness in early childhood', *British Medical Journal* 293 (1986): 303–7.
6. K. Simmer, 'Are iron folate supplements harmful?' *American Journal of Clinical Nutrition* 45 (1987): 122–5.
7. R. M. McClain & J. M. Rohrs, 'Potentiation of the teratogenic effects and altered disposition of diphenylhydrantoin by diet', *Toxicology and Applied Pharmacology* 77 (1985): 86–93.
8. A. Conradt *et al.*, 'Magnesium therapy decreased the rate of intrauterine fetal retardation, premature rupture of membranes and other complications of pregnancy', *Magnesium* 4 (1985): 20–8.
9. See Note 6 in this chapter.
10. L. J. Taper *et al.*, 'Zinc and copper retention during pregnancy: the adequacy of prenatal diets with and without dietary supplementation', *American Journal of Clinical Nutrition* 42 (June 1986): 1184–92.
11. G. Sander *et al.*, 'Hair manganese concentrations in newborns and their mothers', *American Journal of Clinical Nutrition* 41 (1985): 1042–4.
12. R. W. Smithells *et al.*, 'Further experience of vitamin supplementation for prevention of neural tube defect recurrences', *Lancet* 1 (1983): 1027–31. M. J. Seller, 'Periconceptual vitamins and neural tube defects', *Lancet* 1 (1985): 1392–3. J. Wild *et al.*, 'Recurrent neural tube defects, risk factors and vitamins', *Archives of Diseases in Childhood* 61 (1986): 440–9.
13. S. Heller *et al.*, 'Vitamin B status in pregnancy', *American Journal of Clinical Nutrition* 26 (1973): 1339–48.
14. K. Schuster *et al.*, 'Effect of maternal pyridoxine hydrochloride supplementation on the vitamin B_6 status of mother and infant and on pregnancy outcome', *Journal of Nutrition* 114 (1984): 977–88.

15. J. Ellis, 'Vitamin B_6 deficiency in patients with a clinical syndrome including the carpal tunnel defect: biochemical and clinical response to therapy with pyridoxine', *Research Communications in Chemical Pathology and Pharmacology* 13 (1976): 743–50. J. Ellis, 'Clinical results of a crossover treatment with pyridoxine and placebo of the carpal tunnel syndrome', *American Journal of Clinical Nutrition* 32 (1979): 2040–7.

16. J. Marks, 'Critical appraisal of the therapeutic value of alpha-tocopherol', *Vitamins and Hormones* 20 (1962): 573–98.

17. J. Bell *et al.*, 'Perinatal dietary supplementation with a soy lecithin preparation: effects on development of central catecholaminergic neurotransmitter systems', *Brain Research Bulletin* 17 (1986): 189–95.

18. H. Kondo *et. al.*, 'Presence and formation of cobalamin analogues in multivatmin–mineral pills', *Journal of Clinical Investigation* 70 (1982): 889–98.

19. J. A. Mader and I. A. MacDonald, 'Potential mutagenic activity of some vitamin preparations in the human gut', *Applied and Environmental Microbiology* 48 (1984): 902–4.

CHAPTER 3: FROM BIRTH TO SIX MONTHS

1. J. Kumpulainen *et al.*, 'Formula feeding results in lower selenium status than breastfeeding or selenium-supplemented formula feeding: a longitudinal study', *American Journal of Clinical Nutrition* 45 (1987): 49–53.

2. S. Mann & M. F. Picciano, 'Influence of maternal selenium status on human milk selenium concentration and glutathione peroxidase activity', *American Journal of Clinical Nutrition* 46 (1987): 101–9.

3. R. S. Zeiger *et al.*, 'Effectiveness of dietary manipulation in the prevention of food allergy in infants', *Journal of Allergy and Clinical Immunology* 78 (1986): 224–38.

4. J. Azuma, 'Apparent deficiency of vitamin B_6 in typical individuals who commonly serve as normal controls', *Research Communications in Chemical Pathology and Pharmacology* 14 (1976): 343–6.

5. L. Styslinger & A. Kirksey, 'Effects of different levels of vitamin B_6 supplementation of vitamin B_6 concentrations in human milk and vitamin B_6 intakes of breastfed infants', *American Journal of Clinical Nutrition* 41 (1985): 21–31.

6. P. A. Schneider, 'Breast milk jaundice in the newborn: a real entity', *Journal of the American Medical Association* 255 (1986): 3270–4.

7. M. Freundlich *et al.*, 'Infant formula as a cause of aluminium toxicity in neonatal uraemia', *Lancet* 2 (1985): 527–9.

8. P. J. Collipp *et al.*, 'Manganese in infant formulas and learning disability', *Annals of Nutrition and Metabolism* 27 (1983): 488–94.

CHAPTER 4: SIX MONTHS TO A YEAR

1. R. S. Zeiger *et al.*, 'Effectiveness of dietary manipulation in the prevention of food allergy in infants', *Journal of Allergy and Clinical Immunology* 78 (1986): 224–38.
2. E. Pollitt *et al.*, 'Iron deficiency in behavioral development in infants and preschool children', *American Journal of Clinical Nutrition* 43 (1986): 555–65.
3. W. S. Watson *et al.*, 'Oral absorption of lead and iron', *Lancet* 2 (1980): 236–7.
4. M. Fulton *et al.*, 'Influence of blood lead on the ability and attainment of children in Edinburgh', *Lancet* 1 (1987): 1221–5.
5. E. Charney *et al.*, 'Childhood lead poisoning: a controlled trial of the effect of dust control measures on blood lead levels', *New England Journal of Medicine* 309 (1983): 1089–93.
6. A. Kahn *et al.*, 'Insomnia and cow's milk allergy in infants', *Pediatrics* 76 (1985): 880–4.
7. L. Galland, 'Increased requirements for essential fatty acids in atopic individuals: a review with clinical descriptions', *Journal of the American College of Nutrition* 5 (1986): 213–28.
8. A. Cant *et al.*, 'Egg and cow's milk hypersensitivity in exclusively breastfed infants with eczema, and detection of egg protein in breast milk', *British Medical Journal* 291 (1985): 932–4.

CHAPTER 5: AGES 1 TO 5

1. H. J. Roberts, 'Potential toxicity due to dolomite and bone meal', *Southern Medical Journal* 76 (1983): 556–9.
2. M. Bondestam *et al.*, 'Subclinical trace element deficiency in children with undue susceptibility to infection', *Acta Paediatrica Scandinavica* 74 (1985): 515–20.
3. F. A. C. S. Campos *et al.*, 'Effect of an infection on vitamin A status of children as measured by the relative dose response (RDR)', *American Journal of Clinical Nutrition* 46 (1987): 91–4.

CHAPTER 6: NUTRITIONAL FIRST AID TO FIGHT CHILDHOOD ILLNESS

1. R. Anderson *et al.*, 'The effects of increasing weekly doses of ascorbate on certain cellular and humoral immune functions in normal volunteers', *American Journal of Clinical Nutrition* 33 (1980): 71–6.

2. F. A. C. S. Campos, 'Effect of an infection on vitamin A status of children as measured by the relative dose response (RDR)', *American Journal of Clinical Nutrition* 46 (1987): 91–4.

3. C. B. Pinnock *et al.*, 'Vitamin A status in children who are prone to respiratory tract infections', *Australian Paediatric Journal* 22 (1986): 95–8.

4. A. M. El-Hfny, '*Candida albicans* as an important respiratory allergen in the United Arab Republic', *Acta Allergoligica* 23 (1968): 297–302. G. Holti, '*Candida* allergy', in *Symposium on Candida Infections*, ed. H. I. Winner and R. Hurley (London: E. & S. Livingstone Ltd., 1966): 73–81. I. H. Itkin & M. Dennis, 'Bronchial hypersensitivity to extract of *Candida albicans*', *Journal of Allergy* 37 (1966): 187–94. A. Liebeskind, '*Candida albicans* as an allergenic factor', *Annals of Allergy* 20 (1962): 394–6.

5. K. Iwata, 'Toxins reproduced by *Candida albicans*', *Contributions in Microbiology and Immunology* 4 (1977): 77–85.

6. C. O. Truss, 'Tissue injury induced by *Candida albicans*: mental and neurologic manifestations', *Journal of Orthomolecular Psychiatry* 7 (1978): 17–37. C. O. Truss, 'The role of *Candida albicans* in human illness', *Journal of Orthomolecular Psychiatry* 10 (1981): 228–38.

7. S. Wright & J. L. Burton, 'Oral evening primrose seed oil improves atopic eczema', *Lancet* 2 (1982): 1120–2.

8. Consensus Conference – National Institute of Allergy and Infectious Diseases (NIAID) and National Institute of Child Health and Human Development (NICHHD), 'Defined diets and childhood hyperactivity', *Journal of the American Medical Association* 248 (1982): 290–4.

9. I. C. Menzies, 'Disturbed children: the role of food and chemical sensitivities', *Nutrition and Health* 3 (1984): 39–54.

10. R. Gittelman & B. Eskenazi, 'Lead and hyperactivity revisited: an investigation of non-disadvantaged children', *Archives of General Psychiatry* 40 (1983): 827–33.

11. J. Egger *et al.*, 'Controlled trial of oligoantigenic treatment in the hyperkinetic syndrome', *Lancet* 1 (1985): 540–5. J. A. O'Shea & S. F. Porter, 'Double-blind study of children with hyperkinetic syndrome treated with multiallergen extract sublingually', *Journal of Learning Disabilities* 14 (1981): 189–91, 237. E. C. Hughes *et al.*, 'Food sensitivity in attention-deficit disorder with hyperactivity (ADD/HA): a procedure for differential diagnosis', *Annals of Allergy* 49 (1982): 276–80.

12. See Note 11 in this chapter, Hughes citation.

CHAPTER 7: AGES 5 TO 12

1. R. A. Shakman, 'Nutritional influences on the toxicity of environmental pollutants', *Archives of Environmental Health* 28 (1974): 105–13.

2. E. Pollitt *et al.*, 'Iron deficiency in behavioral development in infants and preschool children', *American Journal of Clinical Nutrition* 43 (1986): 555–65.
3. C. A. Clemetson, 'Histamine and ascorbic acid in human blood', *Journal of Nutrition* 110 (1980): 662–8.
4. R. D. Reynolds & C. L. Natta, 'Depressed plasma pyridoxal phosphate concentrations in adult asthmatics', *American Journal of Clinical Nutrition* 41 (1985): 684–8.
5. R. Anderson *et al.*, 'The effects of increasing weekly doses of ascorbate on certain cellular and humoral immune functions in normal volunteers', *American Journal of Clinical Nutrition* 33 (1980): 71–6.
6. F. A. C. S. Campos, 'Effect of an infection on vitamin A status of children as measured by the relative dose response (RDR)', *American Journal of Clinical Nutrition* 46 (1987); 91–4.

CHAPTER 8: AGES 13 TO 17

1. E. W. Rosenberg & B. S. Kirk, 'Acne diet reconsidered', *Archives of Dermatology* 117 (1981): 193–5. A. V. Ratnam & K. Jayaraju, 'Skin diseases in Zambia', *British Journal of Dermatology* 101 (1979): 449–53. E. Bendiner, 'A disastrous trade-off: Eskimo health for white civilization', *Hospital Practice* 9 (1974): 156–89.
2. B. L. Snider & D. F. Dieteman, 'Pyridoxine therapy for premenstrual acne flare', *Archives of Dermatology* 110 (1974): 130–1.
3. S. Ayres Jr & R. Mihan, '*Acne vulgaris* and lipid peroxidation: new concepts in pathogenesis and treatment', *International Journal of Dermatology* 17 (1978): 305–11.
4. G. Michaelsson *et al.*, 'Serum zinc and retinol-binding protein in acne', *British Journal of Dermatology* 96 (1977): 283–90. G. Michaelsson *et al.*, 'A double-blind study of the effect of zinc and oxytetracycline in *Acne vulgaris*', *British Journal of Dermatology* 97 (1977): 561–6. G. Michaelsson *et al.*, 'Effects of oral zinc and vitamin A in acne', *Archives of Dermatology* 113 (1977): 31–6.
5. S. L. Gortmaker *et al.*, 'Increasing pediatric obesity in the United States', *American Journal of the Diseases of Children* 141 (1987): 535–40.
6. A. J. Wittwer *et al.*, 'Nutrient density – evaluation of nutritional attributes of food', *Journal of Nutrition Education* 9 (1977): 26–30, 198.
7. S. Dalvitt-McPhillips, 'A dietary approach to bulimia treatment', *Physiology and Behavior* 33 (1984): 769–75.
8. C. W. M. Wilson, 'Clinical pharmacologic aspects of ascorbic acid', *Annals of the New York Academy of Sciences* 258 (1975): 355–76. R. Hume & E. Weyers, 'Changes in leucocyte ascorbic acid during the common cold',

Scottish Medical Journal 18 (1973): 3–7. P. Roberts *et al.*, 'Vitamin C and inflammation', *Medicine and Biology* 62 (1984): 88–100.

9. W. R. Beisel, 'Single nutrients and immunity', *American Journal of Clinical Nutrition* 35 (supplement) (1982): 417–68. A. B. Carr *et al.*, 'Vitamin C and the common cold: using identical twins as controls', *Medical Journal of Australia* 2 (1981): 411–12. J. Z. Miller *et al.*, 'Therapeutic effect of vitamin C: a co-twin controlled study', *Journal of the American Medical Association* 237 (1977): 248–51.

10. L. E. Mansfield *et al.*, 'Food allergy and adult migraine: double-blind and mediator confirmation of an allergic etiology', *Annals of Allergy* 55 (1985): 126–31. J. Monro *et al.*, 'Migraine is a food-allergic disease', *Lancet* 2 (1984): 719–21. J. Egger *et al.*, 'Is migraine food allergy: A double-blind controlled trial of oligoantigenic diet treatment', *Lancet* 2 (1983): 865–9.

11. B. M. Altura, 'Calcium antagonist properties of magnesium: implications for anti-migraine actions', *Magnesium* 4 (1985): 169–75.

12. McCarrent *et al.*, 'Amelioration of severe migraine by fish oil (N-3) fatty acids', *American Journal of Clinical Nutrition* 41 (abstracts) (1985): 874.

13. H. Bueno & L. Parrish, 'The Bueno-Parrish method (BPM) for diagnosis of intestinal protozoa', *American Journal of Proctocology, Gastroenterology and Colon and Rectal Surgery* 32 (1981): 6, 28.

14. M. Petitpierre *et al.*, 'Irritable bowel syndrome and hypersensitivity to food', *Anals of Allergy* 54 (1985): 538–40. M. A. Smith *et al.*, 'Food intolerance atopy and irritable bowel syndrome', *Lancet* 2 (1985): 1064–6. R. Finn *et al.*, 'Expanding horizons of allergy and the total allergy syndrome', *Clinical Ecology* 3 (1985): 129–31. V. A. Alun-Jones *et al.*, 'Food intolerance: a major factor in the pathogenesis of irritable bowel syndrome', *Lancet* 2 (1982): 1115–17. J. Siegel, 'Inflammatory bowel disease: another possible facet of the allergic diathesis', *Annals of Allergy* 47 (1981): 92–4.

15. D. Ratner *et al.*, 'Milk protein-free diet for nonseasonal asthma and migraine in lactase-deficient patients', *Israel Journal of Medical Sciences* 19 (1983): 806–9.

16. S. Schoenthaler, 'Diet and crime: an empirical examination of the value of nutrition in the control and treatment of incarcerated juvenile offenders', *International Journal of Biosocial Research* 4 (1983): 25–39. S. Schoenthaler & W. Doraz, 'Types of offenses which can be reduced in an institutional setting using nutritional intervention: a preliminary empirical evaluation', *International Journal of Biosocial Research* 4 (1983): 74–84. S. Schoenthaler, 'The Los Angeles Probation Department Diet–Behavior Program: an empirical evaluation of six institutions', *International Journal of Biosocial Research* 5 (1983): 88–98. S. Schoenthaler, 'The Northern California Diet–Behavior Program: an empirical examination of 3000 incarcerated juveniles in Stanislaus County Juvenile Hall', *International Journal of Biosocial Research* 5 (1983): 99–106. S.

Schoenthaler, 'The Alabama Diet–Behavior Program: an empirical evaluation at the Coosa Valley Regional Detention Center', *International Journal of Biosocial Research* 5 (1983): 79–87.
17. D. S. King, 'Can allergic exposure provoke psychological symptoms? A double-blind test', *Biological Psychiatry* 16 (1981): 3–17.

CHAPTER 9: HOW POWER-PACKED NUTRITION CREATES IMMUNITY FOR LIFE

1. M. Alter *et al.*, 'Diet and Multiple Sclerosis', *Archives of Neurology* 31 (1970): 267–70.
2. R. L. Swank, 'Multiple sclerosis: 20 years on a low-fat diet', *Archives of Neurology* 23 (1970): 460–74.
3. Z. Lucas & L. Power, 'Dietary fat aggravates active rheumatoid arthritis', *Clinical Research* 29 (1981): 754a. L. Skoldstam, 'Fasting and vegan diet in rheumatoid arthritis', *Scandinavian Journal of Rheumatology* 15 (1987): 219–21.
4. R. H. Dworkin *et al.*, 'Linoleic acid and multiple sclerosis: a reanalysis of three double-blind trials', *Neurology* 34 (1984): 1441–5. R. H. Dworkin, 'Linoleic acid and multiple sclerosis', *Lancet* 1 (1981): 1153–4.
5. J. M. Kremer *et al.*, 'Effect of manipulation of dietary fatty acids on clinical manifestations of rheumatoid arthritis', *Lancet* 1 (1985): 184–7. J. M. Kremer *et al.*, 'Fish oil fatty acid supplementation in active rheumatoid arthritis: a double-blinded crossover study', *Annals of Internal Medicine* 106 (1987): 497–503.
6. T. H. Lee *et al.*, 'Effect of dietary enrichment with eicosapentaenoic and docosahexaenoic acids on *in vitro* neutrophile and monocyte leukotriene synthesis in rheumatoid arthritis', *New England Journal of Medicine* 312 (1985): 1217–24.
7. See Note 4 in this chapter.
8. D. R. Robinson *et al.*, 'The protective effect of dietary fish oil on murine lupus', *Prostaglandins* 30 (1985): 51–75. W. Yumura *et al.*, 'Dietary fat and immune function – II. Effects on immune complex nephritis (NZB x NZW) F, mice', *Journal of Immunology* 136 (1985): 3864–8. V. E. Kelley *et al.*, 'A fish oil diet rich in eicosapentaenoic acid reduces cyclooxygenase metabolites and suppresses lupus in MRL-lpr mice', *Journal of Immunology* 134 (1985): 1949–59. D. G. Godfrey *et al.*, 'Effects of dietary supplementation on autoimmunity in the MRL/lpr mouse: a preliminary investigation', *Annals of the Rheumatic Diseases* 45 (1986): 1019–24. D. Robinson *et al.*, 'Dietary fish oil reduces progression of established renal disease (NZB x NZW) F, mice and delays renal disease in BXSB and MRL/1 strains', *Arthritis and Rheumatism* 29 (1986): 539–49.

9. V. Johannson *et al.*, 'Nutritional status in girls with juvenile chronic arthritis', *Human Nutrition: Clinical Nutrition* 40c (1986): 57–67. U. Tarp *et al.*, 'Low selenium level in severe rheumatoid arthritis', *Scandinavian Journal of Rheumatology* 14 (1987): 97–100.

10. D. E. Mills & R. P. Ward, 'Effects of essential fatty acid administration on cardiovascular responses to stress in the rat', *Lipids* 21 (1986): 139–42. Kromhoudt *et al.*, 'The inverse relationship between fish consumption and 20-year mortality from coronary heart disease', *New England Journal of Medicine* 312 (1985): 1205–9. B. E. Phillipson *et al.*, 'Reduction of plasma lipids, lipoproteins and apoproteins by dietary fish oils in adults with hyper-lipidemia', *New England Journal of Medicine* 312 (1985): 1210–16. P. G. Norris *et al.*, 'Effect of dietary supplementation with fish oil on systolic blood pressure in mild essential hypertension', *British Medical Journal* 293 (1986): 104–5. J. Iacono *et al.*, 'Dietary fats and the management of hypertension', *Canadian Journal of Physiology and Pharmacology* 64 (1986): 856–62. P. Singer *et al.*, 'Blood pressure and lipid-lowering effect of mackerel and herring diet in patients with mild essential hypertension', *Atherosclerosis* 56 (1985): 223–35.

11. Y. Rayssiguier & E. Gueux, 'Magnesium and lipids in cardiovascular disease', *Journal of the American College of Nutrition* 5 (1986): 507–19.

12. H.-G. Classen, 'Systemic stress magnesium status and cardiovascular damage', *Magnesium* 5 (1986): 105–10.

13. Kromhoudt *et al.*, 'Dietary fibre and ten-year mortality from coronary heart disease, cancer and all causes: The Zutphen Study', *Lancet* 2 (1982): 518–22.

14. J. T. Salonen *et al.*, 'Association between cardiovascular death and myocardinal infarction and serum selenium in a matched-pair longitudinal study', *Lancet* 2 (1982): 175–9.

15. D. P. Rose *et al.*, 'International comparisons of mortality rates from cancer of the breast, ovary, prostate and colon and *per capita* food consumption', *Cancer* 54 (1986): 236;–71

16. R. A. Karmali, 'Fatty acids: inhibition of tumorigenesis', *American Journal of Clinical Nutrition* 45 (1987): 225–9. H. Gabor & S. Abraham, 'Effect of dietary menhaden oil on tumor cell loss and the accumulation of mass of a transplantable mammary adenocarcinoma in mice', *Journal of the National Cancer Institute* 76 (1986): 1223–9. J. J. Jurkowski & W. T. Cave Jr, 'Dietary effects of menhaden oil on the growth and membrane lipid composi-tion of rat mammary tumors', *Journal of the National Cancer Institute* 74 (1985): 1145–50. B. S. Reddy & H. Maruyama, 'Effect of dietary fish oil on azoxymethane-induced colon carcinogenesis in male F344 rats', *Cancer Research* 46 (1986): 3367–70.

17. D. P. Burkitt *et al.*, 'Dietary fibre and disease', *Journal of the American Medical Association* 229 (1974): 1068–73.
18. See Note 13 in this chapter.
19. 'Micronutrient interactions in the prevention of cancer', *Nutrition Reviews* 45 (1987): 139–40. W. C. Willett 'Pre-diagnostic serum selenium and risk of cancer', *Lancet* 1 (1983): 130– 4. M. S. Menkes *et al.*, 'Serum beta-carotene, vitamins A and E, selenium and the risk of lung cancer', *New England Journal of Medicine* 315 (1986): 1250–4. J. T. Salonen *et al.*, 'Risk of cancer in relation to serum concentrations of selenium and vitamins A and E: matched case control analysis of prospective data', *British Medical Journal* 290 (1985): 417–20.

Index